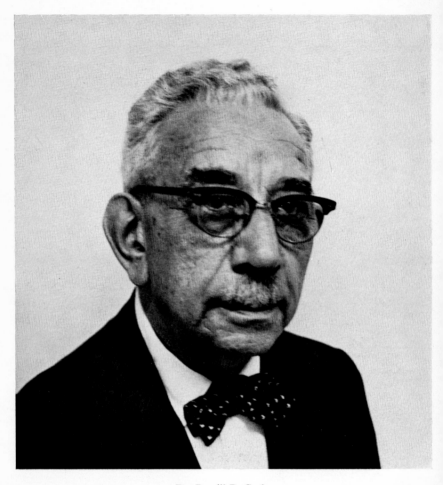

Dr. Burrill B. Crohn.

Frontispiece

Crohn's Disease

Crohn's Disease

James Kyle, *M.Ch. (Belf.), F.R.C.S. (I), F.R.C.S. (Eng.), F.R.C.S. (Edin.)*
Consultant Surgeon, Royal Infirmary, Aberdeen;
Honorary Clinical Senior Lecturer in Surgery,
University of Aberdeen.

THE BRITISH SCHOOL OF OSTEOPATHY
1-4 SUFFOLK STREET, LONDON SW1Y 4HG
TEL: 01-930 9254-8

William Heinemann Medical Books Limited
London

LSNRNJ

First Published 1972

© James Kyle 1972

ISBN 0 433 18900 2

TEXT SET IN 10/11 PT. MONOTYPE TIMES NEW ROMAN, PRINTED BY LETTERPRESS,
AND BOUND IN GREAT BRITAIN AT THE PITMAN PRESS, BATH

Foreword

It is a privilege to be invited to write a foreword to this volume on Regional Enteritis by the author James Kyle of Aberdeen, Scotland. Since the original description of the disease in 1932, this malady has been recognized as having world-wide distribution in practically all climes and countries, and among all classes of society. A voluminous periodical literature describes the medical, surgical and epidemiologic aspects of the disease, but is only fractionally satisfactory.

The need for a comprehensive study, all-inclusive of regional enteritis and colitis has in the last twenty years been lacking. This need is answered in this highly satisfactory and roundly complete volume of the author. Epidemiology, familial incidence, etiology, medical and surgical experience and therapy have all been thoroughly considered. The author's vast experience with the surgical treatment of enteritis is invaluable, as well as the truthful and frank recital of the regrettable rate of post-operative recurrences.

The question still remains open as to whether ulcerative colitis, regional enteritis or granulomatous colitis (so-called Crohn's Disease of the Colon) are affections of this new century, hitherto non-existent, or are they old diseases of many past generations unrecognized till today because of human insufficiencies or because of the former lack of scientific instruments of precision, particularly radiography. If they are really "new" disorders dependent on recent ecological or socio-logical or psychiatric changes, then this present volume with its compre-hensive recital and study of the many etiological factors may offer a clue to this vexatious and interesting quandary.

BURRILL B. CROHN, M.D.

Preface

This book summarizes knowledge about Crohn's disease forty years after the condition was first described. Dr. Burrill B. Crohn has graciously provided the Foreword. Information has accumulated slowly, and there are still large gaps in our understanding of some of the fundamental changes that take place.

The views expressed are those of a surgeon. They are based on the published observations of other workers and on the experience gained from patients with Crohn's disease being studied in north-east Scotland. Different aspects of the disease have been investigated at different times and as a result the numbers of patients mentioned vary slightly between chapters.

The incidence of Crohn's disease appears to be increasing. The late effects of both the disease itself and of empirical forms of treatment are now being recognized. It is hoped that this book will stimulate further research into the cause and cure of Crohn's disease.

JAMES KYLE

74 Rubislaw Den North
    Aberdeen
7 *February* 1972

Contents

Acknowledgements

It is inevitable that in managing and evaluating patients with Crohn's disease, a surgeon must draw on the experience and rely on the advice of colleagues in other specialties. The author is particularly indebted to Dr. L. A. Gillanders, of the Department of Radiodiagnosis, Aberdeen Royal Infirmary, and to Dr. S. W. B. Ewen, of the Department of Pathology, University of Aberdeen, for their assistance so readily given. Professor R. Deans Weir and Miss I. Dingwall-Fordyce advised on statistical problems and Professor J. Swanson Beck helped plan the section on immunology. Dr. P. W. Brunt kindly checked the chapter on medical therapy.

Mr. A. P. R. Aluwihare supplied the electron micrographs in Chapter IV, which are reproduced by permission of the editor of the "Proceedings of the Royal Society of Medicine." The author wishes to thank the editors and publishers of "Gastroenterology", the "Scottish Medical Journal" and the "British Journal of Surgery" for allowing data previously published in their journals to be included in Chapters II, V and X respectively. Figure 1, page 76 appeared in the "Journal of the Royal College of Surgeons of Edinburgh" and is reproduced by courtesy of the editor and Dr. J. F. Fielding. The Department of Medical Illustration, Aberdeen, was most helpful in taking photographs and in providing prints. The figures in Chapter IX are the work of Mr. N. Lukins.

Mrs. C. Smith collected and processed the data on the Aberdeen patients in a very efficient manner. Mrs. J. Kyle corrected all the page proofs.

Finally the author gratefully acknowledges his indebtedness to Miss M. Paterson, who was responsible for the typescript, and to Mr. Owen R. Evans for his assistance in the production of this book.

Chapter I
Historical Introduction

In 1932 Crohn, Ginzburg and Oppenheimer published their classical report on the clinical and pathological entity which today is known as Crohn's disease. Mankind must always have been liable to develop this type of chronic inflammation of the intestines, but the medical profession did not recognize its existence until comparatively recently. Before the middle of the nineteenth century, abdominal operations were not carried out, while autopsies and detailed pathological studies of diseased tissues were uncommon. Although there were rapid advances in surgical, histological and bacteriological techniques after 1850, a full understanding of the types of inflammation within the peritoneal cavity was impeded and rendered difficult by the prevalence of abdominal tuberculosis. Most intestinal lesions that were not clearly either of a neoplastic or of an acute inflammatory nature were likely to be considered tuberculous. However, some of the reports on so-called abdominal tuberculosis published between 1885 and 1930 lack evidence to support this diagnosis. Frequently no mention is made of acid-fast bacilli or caseation.

On re-reading old case histories, in the light of modern knowledge, it seems probable that some of the patients described in the eighteenth and nineteenth centuries had Crohn's disease rather than tuberculosis or other type of inflammation. The young man observed by that pioneer of morbid anatomy, G. B. Morgagni of Forli (1769), had a case history very suggestive of Crohn's disease with perforation. He had been liable to attacks of diarrhoea for most of his life, and at the age of 20 years began getting severe abdominal colic; some blood was passed per rectum. His disease seems to have run a fluctuating course until the patient suddenly became gravely ill and died after 14 days. At autopsy, the terminal ileum and adjacent large bowel were diseased, with inflammation and ulceration on the mucosal surface; perforation had caused a fatal peritonitis. Marked mesenteric adenopathy was noted, and there appears to have been oedema present.

Thirty-seven years later Combe and Saunders described another case to the Royal College of Physicians of London. Again the patient was a young man who "had been for many years troubled with flatulency and complaints in the bowels". He then started to get colicky pain $2\frac{1}{2}$ to 3 hours after eating, and eventually intestinal obstruction supervened. He died on 6th February, 1806, "at which time he was more emaciated than any other person we had ever witnessed". At autopsy there was marked thickening and stenosis of the distal ileum, with three skip areas in the colon. Combe and Saunders postulated that it was the loss of the absorptive function from the lower ileum that caused the marked emaciation.

None of the early reports give any histological evidence to support the clinical and autopsy diagnosis of Crohn's disease. The microscope only became widely used in pathological studies about 120 years ago.

In his monograph on diseases of the stomach and intestinal tract, Abercrombie (1828) described a young girl who conceivably may have had Crohn's disease. Later in the nineteenth century, Moore (1882), in a communication to the Pathological Society of London, gave what is probably the first account of the microscopic appearances in a case of Crohn's disease. Fenwick (1889) in his book on some obscure abdominal diseases recorded the autopsy findings in a women of 27 years: there was enlargement of the lower end of the ileum, with stenosis of the lumen, and the unfortunate patient had at least 2 internal fistulae.

At the beginning of the present century Lartigau (1901), in a study of cases thought to be chronic hyperplastic tuberculosis of the intestine, noted that many of the "tubercles" were only aggregations of lymphoid cells, with one or more giant cells present. There was little tendency to necrotic change and the histological features of tubercle bacilli were often absent. Lartigau clearly realized that there might be other types of granuloma affecting the intestine besides tuberculosis. The following year, Mayo Robson (1902) read a paper to the Clinical Society of London on the surgical treatment of chronic intestinal tuberculosis. From his case reports and illustrations it is almost certain that 3 of his 7 patients had, in fact, Crohn's disease. In 1903, Koch, of Berlin, described two young females with granulomatous lesions in the ileo-caecal region. Tests for tuberculosis were negative. The first of Koch's patients had multiple fistulae and eventually died; his second patient had a successful resection of terminal ileum, with ileo-colic anastomosis. Moynihan, of Leeds, in 1904 carried out a combined excision of rectum in a 28-year-old female for what was probably Crohn's disease. Gradually eminent surgeons such as Moynihan (1907), Robson (1908) and Braun (1909) were realizing that there were non-specific inflammatory lesions in the intestine which could mimic neoplastic disease, and whose resection produced gratifying results. It was about this time at the College of Physicians and Surgeons in New York that Crohn was advised not to read the chapter on the small intestine in Osler's textbook of medicine, because it dealt only with tuberculosis.

The clearest description prior to 1932 of both the clinical and pathological features of Crohn's disease was given by T. Kennedy Dalziel in an address to the 81st Annual Meeting of the British Medical Association on 23rd July, 1913. As surgeon to the Western Infirmary, Glasgow, in 1901 Dalziel had operated on a doctor who, after having had diarrhoea for some time, had then developed subacute obstruction. At laparotomy there was widespread thickening of small and large intestine and no resection was possible. During the following years Dalziel saw 7 more patients with similar chronic inflammation of the intestine that was not tuberculous. He carried out 6 successful resections—of jejunum, mid-ileum, terminal ileum plus caecum (2), transverse colon and sigmoid colon.

Reviewing his cases he pointed out that the most common feature was colicky abdominal pain, often relieved by defaecation. Some blood and mucus might be passed per rectum, the bowel becoming exhausted. Weight loss was noticeable, but there was little elevation of temperature. In one patient he was able to feel a thickened loop of bowel through the abdominal wall; in another he refers to the putty-like resistance felt in the lower abdomen.

Dalziel gave the classic description of the appearances at laparotomy: "The affected bowel gives the consistence and smoothness of an eel in a state of rigor mortis and the glands, though enlarged, are evidently not caseous." His pathologist recognized the transmural nature of the inflammation and stated that the resected specimens constituted "a graded series in which all the stages from acute to chronic may be traced". The earliest changes were said to be congestion and much oedema in the submucosa; later mononuclear cells and the occasional giant cell appeared, in addition to the polymorphonuclear leucocytes.

Although Johnne's disease in cattle had only been recorded in England 6 years earlier (McFadyean, 1907), Dalziel discussed the possible aetiological relationship that might exist between it and the chronic interstitial enteritis from which his patients suffered. The absence of any acid-fast bacilli in the human specimens was noted. In regard to treatment Dalziel did not think that dietetic or medical treatment had any influence on the inflammatory process, and he considered that "only operation can afford relief and then only if the disease be limited". Sixty years later many of the views that Dalziel expressed about Crohn's disease remain substantially correct.

It is surprising that an address given to a large assembly of surgeons did not evoke more interest or stimulate the publication of similar types of case reports from other British medical centres. A quarter of a century was to elapse before Britain made any further significant contribution to the understanding of Crohn's disease. During the two decades following Dalziel's report, nearly all the relevant publications came from German or American hospitals.

In 1914, Läwen described a chronic type of inflammation which involved the appendix, and termed it appendicitis fibroplastica. Twenty-four years later he amended his description and made it clear that originally he was referring to a chronic stenosing type of terminal ileitis. Shortly after the end of the First World War, Tietze (1920) produced a review of all the non-tuberculous intestinal granulomas that had been recorded in the world's literature—281 up to that date. There is little doubt that some of the cases today would be classed as Crohn's disease, but Tietze's review did not define a clinical entity. However, it must have strengthened the belief that there could be lesions other than the prevalent abdominal tuberculosis that could cause thickening and narrowing of the intestine.

Meanwhile in New York, Moschowitz and Wilensky (1923) were seeing patients who had non-specific intestinal granulomas. Their first patient, J.K., who had been troubled by diarrhoea and loss of weight for two years, developed a fistula after an ileal resection in 1918, and had a recurrence in 1920. Like the three other patients with non-tuberculous granuloma of the intestine in this New York series, the patient had had an operation for suppurative appendicitis a short time before a mass appeared. Moschowitz and Wilensky stated: "This lesion can be portioned from the large group of intestinal granulomata." Unfortunately the histories of recent laparotomies suggest that they may have been observing a chronic inflammatory reaction to a foreign-body introduced into the peritoneal cavity. The clinical history and subsequent behaviour of the first patient is very like Crohn's disease, although in the photomicrographs from his resected intestine there are bodies that resemble talc particles. Both Moschowitz and Wilensky were on the attending staff of the Mount Sinai Hospital in New York and their work must have increased interest in and awareness of non-tuberculous intestinal granulomas.

Dr Burrill B. Crohn himself has told the story of how in 1930 he persuaded Dr A. A. Berg at Mount Sinai Hospital to operate on a 17-year-old boy (Crohn, 1967). The patient had suffered from diarrhoea, abdominal pain and a mass, and had intermittent fever. Chest X-ray and the skin tests for tuberculosis then in vogue were negative, and intra-peritoneal oxygen therapy had failed. Resection of ileum was successful. During the next two years Berg and Crohn collected 13 similar cases involving the terminal ileum; many had fistulae from earlier operations. Crohn presented the series at the meeting of the American Medical Association in New Orleans on 13th May, 1932. When it came to publication, Berg modestly declined to have his name in the list of authors and instead suggested that Drs Leon Ginzburg and Gordon Oppenheimer, who were also investigating intestinal granulomas, should join Crohn as co-authors (Crohn, Ginzburg and Oppenheimer, 1932). They described both the clinical and the pathological details of the disease of the terminal ileum much more fully than any previous workers had done. While admitting that the aetiology of the process was unknown, they realized that the disease did not belong to any of the then recognized granulomatous or accepted inflammatory groups.

In this classical series from the Mount Sinai Hospital most of the patients were young, only two being over 40 years; males outnumbered females by almost 2:1. Seven of the patients had had earlier appendicectomies and at some of these operations the inflamed state of the terminal ileum had been noted. There was no evidence of tuberculosis in any of the patients. Crohn and his colleagues distinguished four types of clinical course: (1) acute inflammatory, with a history of only a few days, and at laparotomy a red, soggy oedematous terminal ileum, with prominent glands in the thick mesentery; (2) ulcerative enteritis phase, with diarrhoea, pain, loss of weight and strength going on for months or years; (3) stenotic phase, in which severe colic was associated with a lower abdominal mass; (4) fistulae were often present, 6 of the patients having internal fistulae and others fistulae through appendicectomy scars. They did not encounter any patient with perianal fistulae.

The 1932 paper contained a description of the radiological appearances in the later stages of the disease, and differential diagnosis was considered at some length. The authors' views on treatment were very similar to those expressed 19 years earlier by Dalziel. While advocating resection, they also described Dr Berg's operation of short-circuit with exclusion, and they appreciated that a recurrence might develop. In the discussion that followed the presentation of the paper, several senior clinicians mentioned having seen similar cases. Crohn had called the condition "terminal ileitis"; Bargen, from the Mayo Clinic, suggested the name should be changed to "regional enteritis" as some patients might interpret the use of the adjective "terminal" as meaning that death was imminent. His suggestion was adopted.

The year after Crohn's announcement, Fischer and Lürmann (1933), of Frankfurt-am-Main, described a similar chronic type of lesion in the lower ileum to the German Surgical Congress. Other papers followed in rapid succession during the years before the outbreak of the Second World War. Harris, Bell and Brunn (1933) are usually credited as being the first doctors to identify Crohn's disease in the jejunum, but Dalziel had recorded it in 1913. The latter author had also described the condition in the colon long before Colp's report in 1934.

Indeed there was a strange reluctance for many years to accept the idea that Crohn's disease could affect the colon. A right-sided localized form of colitis had been recorded by Bargen and Weber in 1930. Six years later Crohn and Berg described similar cases, but until the early 1950s gastroenterologists and surgeons tended to regard Crohn's disease as being exclusively a small intestinal granulomatous condition. In 1952 Charles Wells of Liverpool clearly distinguished between ulcerative colitis and what he termed "segmental colitis", and stated his belief that this latter form of colonic lesion was a variant of Crohn's disease. It was characterized by thickening and fibrosis of the colon wall, patchy ulceration of the mucosa and a tendency to spread by "skips". In spite of this clear description, another 8 years were to pass before Lockhart-Mummery and Morson's (1960) paper finally brought general recognition of the colonic involvement. Even then the nomenclature remained in a state of confusion and it was not until the International Congress of Gastroenterology in Prague in 1968 that it was agreed to call the lesion "Crohn's disease of the colon".

Two other events in the history of Crohn's disease merit brief mention. Crohn and his colleagues on histological examination of many of their specimens had seen granulomas composed of epithelioid cells and sometimes giant cells, but they did not regard them as an essential feature. Hadfield, of London, in 1939 produced a detailed study of the histological appearances, and his conclusions were very similar to those of the Mount Sinai Hospital investigators. Unfortunately during the next 20 years his paper was frequently misinterpreted, some pathologists refusing to diagnose Crohn's disease unless granulomas and giant cells were seen. Today all pathologists appreciate that the transmural nature of the inflammation is as important as the type of participating cell.

Crohn's disease had become clearly recognized by doctors, but it was unknown outside the medical profession until President Eisenhower's illness in 1962. Eisenhower had had symptoms intermittently for over 30 years. While he was holding the highest office in the United States of America, a recrudescence necessitated surgical intervention (Heaton, 1964). His operation, described and discussed on American television, first brought Crohn's disease to the attention of the general public.

References

Abercrombie, J. (1828), *Pathological and Practical Researches on Diseases of the Stomach, Intestinal Tract and Other Viscera of the Abdomen*. Edinburgh: Waugh & Innes, p. 238.
Bargen, J. A. and Weber, H. M. (1930), *Surg. Gynec. Obstet.*, **50**, 964.
Braun, H. (1909), *Deutsch. Z. Chir.*, **100**, 1.
Colp, R. (1934), *Surg. Clin. N. Amer.*, **14**, 443.
Combe, C. and Saunders, W. (1813), *Med. Tr. of Coll. Phys. London*, **4**, 16.
Crohn, B. B., Ginzburg, L. and Oppenheimer, G. D. (1932), *J. Amer. med. Ass.*, **99**, 1323.
Crohn, B. B. and Berg, A. A. (1938), *J. Amer. med. Ass.*, **110**, 32.
Crohn, B. B. (1967), *Gastroenterology*, **52**, 767.
Dalzeil, T. K. (1913), *Brit. med. J.*, **2**, 1068.
Fenwick, S. (1889), *Clinical Lectures on Some Obscure Diseases of the Abdomen*. London: Churchill.
Fischer, A. W. and Lürmann, H. (1933), *Arch. für Klin. Chir.*, **177**, 638.
Hadfield, G. (1939), *Lancet*, **2**, 773.
Harris, F. J., Bell, G. H. and Brunn, G. (1933), *Surg. Gynec. Obstet.*, **57**, 637.
Heaton, L. D. (1964), *Ann. Surg.*, **159**, 661.
Koch, J. (1903), *Arch. für Klin. Chir.*, **70**, 891.
Lartigau, A. J. (1901), *J. Exper. Med.*, **6**, 23.
Läwen, A. (1914), *Deutsch. Ztsch. für Chir.*, **129**, 221.
Läwen, A. (1938), *Zentvolbl. für Chir.*, **65**, 911.

Lockhart-Mummery, H. E. and Morson, B. C. (1960), *Gut*, **1**, 87.
McFadyean, J. (1907), *J. Comparat. Path. & Therapeut.*, **20**, 48.
Moore, N. (1882), *Trans. Path. Soc. London*, **34**, 112.
Morgagni, G. B. (1769), *The seats and causes of diseases investigated by anatomy, in Five Books, containing a great variety of dissections and remarks*. London: A. Miller, T. Cadell and Johnston & Payne, Vol. 2, p. 64.
Moschowitz, E. and Wilensky, A. O. (1923). *Amer. J. med. Sci.*, **166**, 48.
Moynihan, B. G. A. (1907), *Edin. med. J.*, **21**, 288.
Robson, A. W. M. (1902), *Trans. Clin. Soc. London*, **35**, 58.
Robson, A. W. M. (1908), *Brit. med. J.*, **1**, 425.
Tietze, A. (1920), *Ergeb. Chir. Orthop.*, **12**, 211.
Wells, C. A. (1952), *Ann. Roy. Coll. Surg. Engl.*, **11**, 105.

Chapter II
Epidemiology

The cause of Crohn's disease is not known. It is by no means certain that there is a single cause. The inflammatory reaction seen by the surgeon and pathologist may represent the intestines' response to several different noxious agents or influences. Crohn's disease does not occur spontaneously in lower animals. Attempts to produce chronic lesions in them have not been successful. The only animal available for study is man.

In human beings many diseases only become established because of a combination of factors. The soil must be prepared before the aetiological agent or agents can trigger off the pathological process. Some of the preparing factors such as geography, race and heredity apply to large groups of people and will have been operative long before any individual patient is born; together they are sometimes referred to as the macrocosm. However, the potential patient does have some say in his mode of living, the food he eats, his place of residence and whether he remains single or gets married; these personal characteristics, social and domestic factors constitute the microcosm. In an unfortunate individual who happens to have a malign combination of these various factors, some comparatively trivial incident such as a small abrasion of the intestinal mucosa releasing intracellular protein may be enough to precipitate the start of a prolonged and disabling disease.

In helping to elucidate the causation of chronic conditions such as Crohn's disease, epidemiological studies perform two useful functions: they highlight the preparatory factors and may considerably narrow the field of search for the precipitating agent. A good epidemiological survey of a community is difficult to organize and time-consuming to carry out. The protocols for the survey should: (a) define the geographical limits and the population at risk; (b) describe the methods of ascertainment used; (c) state the diagnostic criteria employed; (d) list any exclusions from the survey, e.g. visitors to the community, or students or soldiers who are not a permanent part of it. The number of cases available for study needs to be reasonably large so as to permit meaningful statistical analyses to be performed on the results. A prospective study, with personal interviews of patients, is better than retrospective examination of case records.

Inevitably these desiderata are very rarely met. As far as Crohn's disease is concerned there is only one published study, that of Norlen *et al.* (1970) from Central Sweden, which meets most of these requirements.

However there are many reports that do provide some useful information. They may be considered in three groups. The first group consists of many reports, often of only small series of patients, coming from countries in all parts of the world. They are considered along with information that the author has obtained from experienced surgeons and pathologists working in countries from which no reports have come. Taken together they provide a good picture of the global distribution of Crohn's disease and, less accurately, of possible racial influences.

In the second group there are larger series of patients collected by one person, by a special service, such as the Veterans' Administration service, by large private clinics and also the national survey of Gjone *et al.* (1966) from Norway. In general they do not represent a detailed scrutiny of a fixed community. Respected institutions and clinicians can attract patients from far afield. However, these reports do allow conclusions to be drawn about age and sex distribution and religion.

The third group—and final part of this chapter—consists of the Swedish epidemiological survey (Norlen *et al.*, 1970) and the comparable investigation carried out in north-east Scotland between 1955 and 1969. (Kyle, 1971). The two surveys were performed independently and without knowledge of each other; for brevity they will frequently be referred to as the Uppsala and the Aberdeen series respectively. Most of the views and conclusions expressed in later chapters of this book are based on the experience gained with the 166 patients from the Aberdeen series.

Global Distribution

Australasia

During 8 years as a surgeon in Suva, Fiji, de Beaux (1970) did not see a single case of Crohn's disease in a non-European. The population of 300,000 that the War Memorial Hospital serves is divided almost equally between Fijians and Indians. It has been suggested (Norlen *et al.*, 1970) that the disease is rare in the Maoris of New Zealand on the basis of the paper published by Wigley and Maclaurin (1962). In fact these authors did not study Crohn's disease, only ulcerative colitis, no case of which was found in Maoris in the Wellington area.

The continent of Australia has a population of approximately 12 million, or rather less than one-quarter of that in Britain. There is a general impression that Crohn's disease is uncommon (Fone, 1966) but to date no epidemiological survey has been undertaken. The principal hospitals in the two largest cities have only recorded comparatively small series. In Melbourne, Fone (1966) collected 41 patients, 22 being female and 19 male. There was a more marked female preponderence among the 30 patients with Crohn's disease of the colon studied by McGovern and Goulston (1968) in Sydney. The majority of Australians are of British ancestry and standards of medical care are similar to those in Britain (the method of payment is different). It is therefore surprising that larger series of patients with Crohn's disease have not been reported. In their absence it must be assumed that the condition is somewhat less prevalent than in Britain.

Asia

Gastroenterology is a major speciality in Japan, and patients with regional ileitis have been reported from that country. One of the largest series is that of Yamase *et al.* (1967). They collected 542 cases published in Japanese journals during a 15-year period. More than 70 per cent were of acute type; no fistulae and no recurrences were seen. Their review provided no histological confirmation of the diagnosis. In 1966 the author was privileged to attend a meeting of the Japanese Surgical Society in Hokkaido at which a paper on "Acute Ileitis" was presented. It transpired that this was a parasitic infestation prevalent on the west coast of Hokkaido, caused by Anisakis larvae and transmitted by pollack and similar fish caught off the coast (Ishikura *et al.*, 1967). With its rapidly rising standard of living and industrialization it would be surprising if Crohn's disease did not occur in Japan—assuming that the modern way of life plays some role in aetiology. However, until more studies specifically excluding other causes of enteric infection and infestation have been published it may be safer to regard the identity between the Japanese and the Western forms of Crohn's disease as "not proven".

At the Queen Mary Hospital in Hong Kong during the years 1964–1968, Gibson (1970) encountered only one case of Crohn's disease in a Chinese patient. The hospital serves a population of approximately one million. At Chiengmai in the north west corner of Thailand some of the medical staff are or have been trained by American graduates, principally from the University of Illinois. They are willing to admit that a few patients with Crohn's disease have been diagnosed. Across the border in Burma, although the influence of British medicine remains strong (Harrison, 1970), Crohn's disease is virtually unknown. The same is true in Nepal, no cases having been detected at the Bir Hospital in Katmandu (Sharma, 1966).

Many of the beds in general surgical wards in teaching hospitals in northern India are filled with patients suffering from abdominal tuberculosis. It would be very difficult to separate patients with Crohn's disease from them. However, there is at least one good, although generally overlooked report on Crohn's disease from Calcutta. Among the teeming millions in that city, Gupta and his colleagues (1962) diagnosed and operated on 44 patients, 28 being females. Their results put to shame those being obtained in many European and American centres.

At Shiraz, in southern Iran, Crohn's disease has never been recognized. Many of the staff at the Saadi and Nemazi Hospitals are Western-trained. There is an active interest in intestinal conditions (Saidi, 1970) and the absence of Crohn's disease from their records refutes the suggestion that the incidence of the disease is directly related to the number of doctors who have studied in Britain and America. In Turkey, Aktan (1970) saw 9 patients with Crohn's disease among 17,000 people attending the Gastroenterology Clinic of the Ankara University Hospital, during the years 1965 to 1969. Five of the 9 patients were females and their ages ranged from 27 to 40 years.

Probably the most interesting omission in the global epidemiology of Crohn's disease is the absence of any detailed survey in Israel. Jews are said to be more likely to develop the disease than are those belonging to other religions, certainly in the United States (Acheson, 1960). However, in Jerusalem, Crohn's disease is uncommon in Jews who have migrated from southern Europe or America and practically unknown among those who have come from elsewhere in Asia and North Africa (Rozen, 1970). A good survey in Israel is clearly needed.

Africa
Most of the nations on the African continent are steadily developing their medical services. Until now details about the incidence of particular diseases have been difficult to obtain, and this has certainly been true of Crohn's disease. During 15 years in Malawi (then Nyasaland) Baird (1970) never saw a case of Crohn's disease. Cumming-Smith (1970) had a similar completely negative experience in Tanzania (then Tanganyika), but Kibaya (1946) did report one possible case from East Africa. In South Africa the disease does develop occasionally in Europeans in Cape Province (Brom *et al.*, 1968); it is rarely seen in Bantus in the Transvaal (Girault *et al.*, 1969) and almost never in Bantus in Natal (Baker, 1970).

Europe
Language difficulties make an assessment of the incidence of Crohn's disease in Russia and Eastern Europe difficult. From the few reports and small series published it would seem that the disease is uncommon (Kubicki, 1964); the incidence may be similar to that in Turkey.

Maratka and his colleagues (1968) in Czechoslovakia have published numerous papers, mainly dealing with Crohn's disease of the colon, which appears to be relatively common in Bohemia. In presenting epidemiological studies it seems advisable to deal separately with small bowel and with large bowel granulomatous disease. They may be the same condition. On the other hand they may differ in the way that duodenal ulceration differs from gastric ulceration—considering these two lesions as one, "peptic ulceration", did nothing to help elucidate their respective aetiologies. Yovanovich (1961) has reported a series of cases of Crohn's disease from Jugoslavia.

In Italy (Ferrara and Balbo, 1966) and Germany (Morl, 1966) the reports mostly come from one hospital and show a slight male preponderance. It is unfortunate that no epidemiological survey seems to have been carried out in Austria or Germany because Monk *et al.* (1969) believed that Americans whose ancestors came from those countries might be more susceptible to Crohn's disease. In Western Europe, excluding Scandinavia and the British Isles, the only large series of patients is that collected in Louvain, Belgium (Vantrappen *et al.*, 1966). Although geographically close to Britain, the sex ratio is different in the two countries, males outnumbering females by 2:1 in Belgium. Apart from this the disease pattern is similar.

Crohn's disease is common in Britain and in Scandinavia. Much original work has been done in Denmark, Sweden and Norway. The epidemiological results are considered in more detail on page 17 but it is worth noting the unexplained disparity between the incidence of 0·26 per 100,000 population per annum in Norway and the 2·5 figure for Central Sweden (Table 1).

Table 1

Incidence of Crohn's disease in five countries
(per 100,000 of population per annum)

Country	Region or group	Incidence	Authors
U.S.A.	Baltimore: whites	1·35	
	non-whites	0·04	Mendeloff *et al.*, 1966
	non-Jews	0·8	
England	Oxford	0·8	Evans *et al.*, 1965
	Leeds	3·5	de Dombal, 1970
Scotland	Aberdeen	2·2	Kyle, 1971
Norway	National series	0·26	Gjone *et al.*, 1966
Sweden	Uppsala	2·5	Norlen *et al.*, 1970

It has been stated that Crohn's disease is rare in Ireland (Edwards, 1964). No survey to confirm or refute this contention has been carried out to date. From an aetiological point of view it is interesting that sarcoidosis is relatively much more common in Irish immigrants in the London area than it is in the native English (Hall *et al.*, 1969). Few cases of Crohn's disease are seen in Iceland (Jonasson, 1970), a country which has close ties with Scandinavia and Scotland and which would be very suitable for an epidemiological survey.

The Americas

From evidence appearing in local medical journals and from personal enquiries made by the author, the incidence of Crohn's disease in Argentina apparently is similar to that recorded in Australia and in the Caucasians in South Africa. Some cases are encountered in Santiago de Chile, but Crohn's disease may be rarer in Peru and Colombia—detailed information is lacking. The considerable admixture of Amerindian,

Caucasian and African blood in the western parts of South America would make some epidemiological data unusually difficult to interpret.

Several reports have come from Central America. Martinez (1968) described 8 cases seen in hospitals in Santa Ana, El Salvador, during a period of 22 years; there was only one female in the series. Jinch *et al.* (1967) collected 22 Mexican patients who had been treated in 9 hospitals, principally in Mexico City in the 13 years up to 1966. Seventeen of the patients were females; most patients had developed the disease in the 4th decade of life, and the average age was decidedly higher than in other published reports. Crohn's disease was commoner among Jews than among non-Jews in Mexico; it was diagnosed as often in public hospitals as in private institutions. Among over 300,000 hospital admissions in Havana, Cuba, Chacon (1966) was able to find only 11 patients with Crohn's disease—a low hospital admission rate. He reviewed 40 other patients from the Cuban medical literature. Females outnumbered males by 3:2; very few people of African or oriental ancestry were affected.

The greatest concentration of cases of Crohn's disease in North America is in the north-east (Mendeloff *et al.*, 1966), in the Baltimore–Boston–Cleveland triangle. This is the region with the highest population density in the United States and includes New York City. Crohn's disease has been reported from almost every state in the Union. However, on a population basis it is less common in the southern states, probably because of the higher proportion of negroes there. The condition is comparatively rare in negroes in North America, but does occur in them (Ratzloff and Jacobs, 1970). The incidence is almost certainly considerably greater than among the people of tropical Africa. Negroes are prone to develop sarcoidosis. In contrast to Crohn's disease, sarcoidosis occurs most frequently in the south-eastern part of the United States, and nearly half the patients are negroes (Gentry *et al.*, 1955). It is said that Crohn's disease is uncommon in Wisconsin, the dairy state (Warthin, 1968); the reason is not known. From Canada there are series reported from all the states between Quebec and British Columbia. The pattern of Crohn's disease is similar to that south of the 49th parallel. The disease is believed to be rare in Eskimos (Gilbert and Sartor, 1964).

From this global survey it can be concluded that Crohn's disease is most common in north-west Europe and in the north-east part of North America. Although most of their ancestors will have come from these high-risk areas, Caucasians living in the Southern Hemisphere are less liable to develop Crohn's disease. This is true even in cities with populations of over one million, such as Sydney and Buenos Aires. The average age of the population in tropical countries is markedly lower than in temperate zones, and Crohn's disease most often occurs in young adults. Nevertheless, Crohn's disease is rare in Asia and Africa. Whether this discrepancy is accounted for by racial factors, or the mode of living, by the predominance of other diseases or by poor diagnostic facilities and documentation is not known at the present time.

Larger Series

More than 1,200 patients with Crohn's disease have been treated at the Mount Sinai Hospital, New York. As in other centres in North America there has been a slight excess of males over females. The percentage of females in several large American and European series is shown in Table 2. In the second edition of their book Crohn and Yarnis (1958)

Table 2

Sex distribution in Crohn's disease: percentage of female patients in 10 large series

Country	Region or clinic	Percentage female	Authors
U.S.A.	Mount Sinai Hospital	43	Crohn *et al.*, 1958
	Mayo Clinic	44	Van Patter *et al.*, 1954
	Lahey Clinic	48	Colcock *et al.*, 1960
Belgium	Louvain	50	Vantrappen *et al.*, 1966
England	London	54	Edwards, 1964
	Birmingham	52	Fielding, 1970
	Leeds	54	de Dombal, 1970
Scotland	Aberdeen	64	Kyle, 1971
Norway	National series	50	Gjone *et al.*, 1966
Sweden	Uppsala	47	Norlen *et al.*, 1970

stated that nearly 40 per cent of their patients, then numbering 676, were aged between 20 and 30 years. At the time of publication large bowel involvement was not so frequently recognized; it is this form of the disease that may increase the incidence in later life. At that time (1958) Crohn and Yarnis challenged the widely held belief that the disease was commoner in Jews. They stated that any race could be affected and that Jews were not particularly susceptible.

However, two years later Acheson (1960) published the results of a detailed investigation into the incidence of ulcerative colitis and Crohn's disease in United States veterans (ex-servicemen). Out of 698 patients with regional enteritis 8·8 per cent professed the Jewish faith, a proportion four times as high as in a control sample of the hospital population. This high proportion existed irrespective of which part of the United States the patients had been born in, and was equally true for veterans of both World Wars and the Korean War. However, even higher proportions of Jews have been recorded. In the Mayo Clinic series (van Patter *et al.*, 1954) 25 per cent of the patients were Jewish, and in the Harper Hospital, Detroit, 43 out of 100 patients were Jews (Ruble *et al.*, 1957). As Acheson (1960) points out, neither of these institutions is a Jewish foundation.

Six hundred patients first attended the Mayo Clinic with Crohn's disease in the years up to 1950; 44 per cent were females. The annual incidence rose steadily until 1941. Thereafter the rate of increase slowed. The annual attendances were maximal in the war years 1943 and 1944; they then declined slightly. Warthin (1968) has reported that Crohn's disease is rare in combat zones in wartime, possible due to the quality of the food. Crohn's disease started in 38 per cent of the Mayo Clinic patients during the 3rd decade of life.

Other large series have been published from such centres as the Cleveland Clinic (Daffner and Brown, 1958) and the Lahey Clinic, Boston (Colcock and Vansant, 1960). Like the Mayo Clinic in Minnesota, these private institutions attract patients from far afield. Their disease statistics do not represent the incidence of disease in a limited, local and static community.

The Baltimore survey published by Mendeloff (1966), Monk (1969) and their associates was the first one in America to clearly define the population studied and the diagnostic criteria that were adhered to. In many respects it was similar to the epidemiological survey carried out in the Oxford region of England by Evans and Acheson (1965). In both Crohn's disease played the minor part in a study where ulcerative colitis was the major interest. Both studies were retrospective, patients were not seen and there was no follow-up. In Baltimore City, 95 patients with Crohn's disease had attended hospital during the 1960–1963 period. They were compared with matched hospital controls. The incidence (first hospitalization) of Crohn's disease per 100,000 of the white population per annum was 1·35 whereas for the coloured population the corresponding figure was only 0·04. When Jews were compared with non-Jews the figures were 7·0 and 0·8 respectively; the latter figure is identical with that in Oxford. A higher proportion of Jews developed Crohn's disease before the age of 35 years compared to non-Jews. The families of Jewish patients had been in the United States longer than those of control patients. Crohn's disease was commoner in those with an urban rather than a rural background and in Baltimore white-collar workers and the better educated were more likely to develop the disease than were those at the lower end of the socio-economic scale. More patients remained unmarried compared to the controls, and Monk *et al.* (1969) speculate on whether or not this might have been due to a chronic illness in young adult life reducing the chances of matrimony.

Most of the data in Evans' and Acheson's (1965) Oxford survey relates to ulcerative colitis. They accepted only 24 patients as having Crohn's disease in a population of 264,000 during a 10-year period to the end of 1960. The annual incidence was thus 0·8 per 100,000 and the prevalence rate 9 per 100,000. Crohn's disease of the colon was not widely recognized before 1960; some of the patients that the Oxford workers termed "mixed forms" would now be classified as Crohn's disease. With such small numbers to investigate, the value of the Oxford study of the epidemiology of Crohn's disease is strictly limited. However, it did prove the reliability of the Records Departments in British hospitals and the accuracy of ascertainment.

There are three series of 300 or more patients collected in England over periods of about 30 years. That of Edwards (1969) was partly personal and partly a King's College Hospital, London, series. Cooke accumulated his 300 cases in the Birmingham region (Fielding, 1970a), while there has been an active interest in Crohn's disease at the Leeds General Infirmary for many years (Armitage and Wilson, 1950; de Dombal, 1970).

In these three English series there is a slight excess of females over males; the female preponderance is even greater in Scotland. Leeds and the surrounding area are highly industrialized. de Dombal (1970) has been able to calculate the incidence rate in the most recent period as being 3·5 per 100,000 per year. The incidence among Jews in Baltimore was twice this figure, but apart from that, the Leeds incidence is the highest that has been reported from a community.

The occurrence of Crohn's disease and ulcerative colitis within families has been described, although the underlying mechanism and significance are not clear. Their coexistence does suggest an aetiological relationship. Kirsner and Spencer (1963) reviewed the literature on familial occurrence from the first report by Lewisohn (1938). Among their own 185 patients with Crohn's disease at the University of Chicago hospitals, there were 12 relatives with the same disease and 9 with ulcerative colitis. This is a familial incidence of 11 per cent. The same generation was most often affected; two-thirds of the familial cases were in brothers, sisters or cousins although many of them lived far apart. The familial tendency was greater in families of Jewish origin. In London, Lennard-Jones (1968) found a first-degree relative affected in 6 per cent of 145 cases at St Mark's and the Central Middlesex Hospitals. These two hospitals and Kirsner's clinic in Chicago are well known for their interest in intestinal diseases. However, Crohn recorded a familial incidence of only 2 to 3 per cent. Edwards (1969) at King's College Hospital, London, had 4 pairs of brothers or brothers and sisters afflicted with Crohn's disease in a series of 302 patients. He did not consider genetic influences to be important in predisposing to Crohn's disease. In north-east Scotland, out of 166 patients there has been one instance of two members (mother and son) being affected by Crohn's disease, although three other patients had one parent with ulcerative colitis. Aggregation of cases within a few families does not necessarily prove a genetic relationship although the genetic influence must be stronger than environment when affected members of a family are living far apart. It seems probable that there is some genetically determined susceptibility to an unknown precipitating agent. Classical Mendelian ratios are not found in affected families (Almy and Sherlock, 1966) and probably the gene responsible is of low penetrance and not sex-linked.

In the East End of London, Wright (1970) has recently observed a seemingly remarkable clustering of cases of Crohn's disease. Eight patients who were not related to each other all lived within a small area. The number of years during which these cases arose is not known, and consequently the effect of environment cannot be accurately assessed. Clustering of cases has not been noted by other workers.

The retrospective study that Gjone *et al.* (1966) carried out in Norway (population 3,500,000) was on a national basis covering the years 1956 to 1963 inclusive. Altogether 173 cases were reported to them; they excluded nearly 100 of these but do not describe the diagnostic criteria that these patients failed to meet. The mean annual incidence was only 0·26 per 100,000. It was 0·17 in the first 4-year period and doubled in the second 4 years. There was no sex difference, no regional variation and no patient below 14 years of age. The low incidence in Norway is surprising when it is compared to the results in the adjacent part of central Sweden. Many of the Norwegian patients would have been children or teenagers during the privations of the wartime occupation. The annual incidence in the country has now risen to 1 per 100,000 (Gjone, 1970).

Aberdeen and Uppsala Series

The epidemiological survey in north-east Scotland was conducted during the years 1955–1969 inclusive, and was prospective from 1960 onwards. All patients except 4 who had died before 1960 have been seen by the author and all have been followed up. The area of the study was the City of Aberdeen (population 185,000) and the 4 adjacent counties (population 257,000), the hospital services for which are provided by the teaching hospitals of the University of Aberdeen. Geographically the area is bounded by sea on the east and north, while to the west and south-west mountains, separate it from the remainder of Scotland. Thus it is clearly defined and compact. The hospital buildings are new and the University contains the oldest Faculty of Medicine in the English-speaking world (established 1494). Consequently very few people indeed seek medical advice outside the region—far less than the 5 per cent accepted by Evans and Acheson (1965) in Oxford.

As in the Oxford survey, the Central Records Department for the region proved the most reliable method of ascertainment. In addition, all radiological examinations of the gastrointestinal tract are reported to one department and all pathological specimens are dealt with in the University's laboratory. All colons that had been resected for ulcerative disease since 1955 were re-examined. Every year each physician and surgeon was asked to notify any possible, probable or proven case of Crohn's disease. So far as is known every patient was in hospital at some time during the study period. Being a chronic disease it is most unlikely that any patient lucky enough not to require admission could avoid having an X-ray or biopsy for 15 years.

The diagnosis of Crohn's disease rests on 4 main pillars—(1) clinical picture—colic, diarrhoea, weight loss and, in about 40 per cent, a palpable mass; (2) radiological appearances (page 91); (3) macroscopic appearances at laparotomy (page 48); (4) transmural inflammation on histological examination, with granulomas and giant cells in 65 to 70 per cent of specimens. At least 2 of these criteria had to be met before a case was accepted; the behaviour of the lesion over a period of time was important in arriving at a decision in some cases.

Visitors, students and others who had only spent a few weeks or months in north-east Scotland were excluded. Nine patients who had first developed their disease and received part of their treatment elsewhere and 10 cases of so-called "acute Crohn's disease" are not included in the epidemiological survey, but are considered in Chapter V.

Norlen *et al.* (1970) carried out their investigation during the years 1956 to 1967 on a similar mixed urban and rural population of 412,000, centred on Uppsala. Their methods and criteria were essentially similar to those employed in Aberdeen, except that their study was retrospective and they did not separate Crohn's disease of the colon from that of the small bowel.

Results

Up to the end of 1969 in the Aberdeen area 166 patients developed or were treated for Crohn's disease. In 133 cases the small bowel was the principal site of involvement, while in 33 cases (20 per cent) it was the large bowel that was predominantly affected (Kyle, 1971.)

Incidence

In 16 patients Crohn's disease had started before 1955, and they are therefore omitted from calculations of annual incidence, as are those starting in 1969—some may still await detection. The Aberdeen incidence rates are based on 134 patients whose date of onset was in the 14-year period to the end of 1968. Date of onset was chosen instead of date of diagnosis because it eliminates one variable—the fallibility of the medical profession. In Uppsala there were 123 patients in 12 years. The end of 1961 marks the mid-point of both series. The change in the annual incidence per 100,000 during the two 7-year periods in Aberdeen and the two 6-year periods in Uppsala is shown in Table 3. There has been an increase in both series, but whereas in Uppsala the increase in the second period was mainly in younger males, in Aberdeen it was more marked in older females. During the 14 years in the Aberdeen area the incidence averaged 2·2 per 100,000 per year. Acute suppurative appendicitis is about 80 times more common.

Table 3

*Incidence of Crohn's disease during the two halves of the Aberdeen
and the Uppsala surveys (per 100,000 per annum)*

Sex	Aberdeen		Uppsala	
	1955–1961	*1962–1968*	*1956–1961*	*1962–1967*
Male	1·4	1·6	1·8	3·4
Female	1·9	3·0	1·8	2·8

Prevalence

To obtain the prevalence of a chronic disease on a certain date, the numbers of people who died and who emigrated are subtracted from the total number diagnosed during the study period. The resulting figure is divided by the population at risk, the prevalence rate being expressed per 100,000 of population. At the end of 1967 in the Uppsala region the rate was 27, while in Aberdeen at the end of 1968 it was 32·5 per 100,000.

Sex

In the Aberdeen series 63 per cent of the patients were females. However, in Uppsala females only accounted for 43 per cent of the total. The reason for the large proportion of females in Scotland is not known, but a variety of gastrointestinal diseases, such as duodenal ulceration, intussusception and diverticulitis are relatively commoner in the female sex in Scotland than they are in England (Kyle and Blair, 1965).

Age at Onset

For the 166 patients in the Aberdeen series, the decade of onset is shown in Table 4 for males and for females, together with the corresponding population at risk (to nearest thousand; 1961 census). It is

Table 4

Age of onset for males and females in north-east Scotland

Age at onset (years)	Females		Males	
	No. of patients	*Population*	*No. of patients*	*Population*
0–9	—	36,000	—	37,000
10–19	19	35,000	12	36,000
20–29	26	29,000	16	27,000
30–39	13	29,000	14	28,000
40–49	19	29,000	7	26,000
50–59	13	30,000	2	26,000
60–69	6	24,000	5	17,000
70–79	8	14,000	4	10,000
80+	2	6,000	—	3,000
Total	106	232,000	60	210,000

2

obvious from this table that the chances of developing Crohn's disease are greatest in the 3rd decade of life. Considering the relatively small number of people aged 70 years and over in any community, there is a second minor peak in the incidence rate towards the end of life. Among 20,000 elderly females there were no less than 10 cases of Crohn's disease diagnosed up to 1969. Although presented in a slightly different manner and covering the years 1960 to 1965 only, the Uppsala data points to similar conclusions—peak incidence between 20 to 29 years of age, and a minor peak, mainly in females, after 70 years. The main peak only became obvious during the second 6 years of their study. It will be noted that in Aberdeen there was no case of Crohn's disease under the age of 10 years; in Sweden there were 2 such young patients.

Site of Disease

Eighty per cent of the Aberdeen series (133 out of 166) were in the small intestine, almost always in the distal ileum. In some of these patients there was involvement of the adjacent part of the caecum and in a few instances a "contact" lesion had developed on the apex of the sigmoid loop. In the 33 patients classified as colonic, the disease had first started and mostly remained confined to the colon, often having "skip" lesions therein. A few patients later developed disease in the terminal ileum. The age of onset of small bowel and of colonic Crohn's disease is given in Table 5. There were just as many cases of Crohn's disease of

Table 5

Age at onset of Crohn's disease of the small bowel and of the colon

Age at onset (years)	Small bowel No. of patients	Colon No. of patients	Population (1961)
0–9	—	—	73,000
10–19	25	6	71,000
20–29	39	3	56,000
30–39	25	2	57,000
40–49	20	6	55,000
50–59	9	6	56,000
60–69	8	3	41,000
70–79	6	6	24,000
80+	1	1	9,000
Total	133	33	442,000

the colon in the 8th decade as at any earlier period of life, even though the number of people at risk is very much smaller. Most of these elderly colonic patients were females. No comparable data regarding site is given in the Uppsala data.

Place of Residence

The Baltimore workers (Mendeloff *et al.*, 1966) have suggested that Crohn's disease was more prevalent in urban dwellers than in people from rural areas. Norlen *et al.* (1970) were unable to detect any difference in incidence between city and country in central Sweden. However in north-east Scotland there was a marked difference. There were 92 cases within the city boundary of Aberdeen (population 185,000) compared to 74 in the larger surrounding rural area (population 257,000) which includes some small towns and suburban districts. Relatively fewer males were affected both in the city and the country areas; the difference in the country is statistically highly significant (Table 6). There were also relatively few females in country areas, but the difference was less marked.

Table 6

Incidence by place of residence

Sex	Residence	Incidence per 100,000	Significance
Male	Country	17·5	$X^2 = 13·24$
	City	44·5	$p < 0·001$
Female	Country	39·3	$X^2 = 7·27$
	City	54·0	$p < 0·01$

Marital Status

In north-east Scotland 35 per cent of the population over the age of 10 years is unmarried. Among the 166 patients with Crohn's disease 31 per cent were unmarried when the disease began. Six of the females are known to have married since the onset, and another has married for the second time. Without direct questioning, it is not possible to state how many of the surviving males have changed their marital status from the onset of their disease up to the end of 1970. However, this Scottish experience is clearly at variance with the less happy matrimonial prospects of the Baltimore patients.

Social Grade

The occupation of the family breadwinner was known for 164 out of the 166 Scottish patients. Because of the relatively small numbers available for analysis, grades I and II (white-collar) were grouped together as were grades IV and V (the unskilled and semi-skilled); skilled workers occupied an intermediate group. When these groups were compared with the corresponding population groups from the 1961 census, there was only a slight difference detectable. In Baltimore white-collar workers were more often affected, but in Aberdeen Crohn's disease was relatively uncommon in this group. The Swedish workers did not study social grades. It would be interesting to know if during a patient's lifetime the social grade of his family had altered; Monk *et al.* (1970) doubt if this is of any importance.

Hereditary Factors

The low familial incidence in the Aberdeen series has been mentioned (page 16); a son developed Crohn's disease 20 years after his mother had had a resection for the same condition. Mother and son is the most common type of parent–child familial relationship in Crohn's disease. In Uppsala too, only one family had more than one member affected; there was the possibility of a cousin of another patient having Crohn's disease. It therefore seems that in Sweden and Scotland the hereditary influence is weak. However, there probably is a tendency both for the incidence of the disease in the relatives of propositii to be underestimated and for unaffected members of a family not to be recorded at all. No Jews appeared in either series.

Blood Group

The distribution of the blood groups in 134 of the Aberdeen patients was practically identical with that in 5,000 normal blood donors in the region. Edwards (1969) noted that 58 per cent of his male patients belonged to blood group O. It is not clear whether the people he contrasted them with were derived from the same population—a very important point in blood group studies. The data were not analysed for Rh or other blood group systems in the Aberdeen patients; they merit investigation in the future.

Interpretation

An epidemiological survey can be brought to a successful conclusion by careful planning and hard work. With increasing experience, mistakes become fewer and more data is produced. The real difficulty comes in attempting to interpret the data. Speculation can sometimes run riot until suddenly it is confronted by irreconcilable fact. Theories must be abandoned, but new lines of investigation then suggest themselves, and must be tackled.

The global distribution of Crohn's disease resembles that of diverticulitis (Kyle *et al.*, 1967); this does not necessarily imply an aetiological relationship. Indeed it is unlikely as the majority of patients with Crohn's disease are less than 40 years old whereas colonic diverticula do not appear before that age. Crohn's disease is rare in those parts of the world where tuberculosis is still common. It has been suggested that the intestinal disease could be an abnormal immunological reaction resulting from lack of exposure to *Mycobacterium tuberculosis* (Fielding, 1970b). However in Western Europe and North America both diseases were encountered for 20 years after 1932.

The low incidence of Crohn's disease among coloured people in the United States does suggest that a racial factor plays some role. These coloured people eat the same processed food and are subjected to the same atmospheric pollution as the Caucasians around them. Admittedly socio-economic circumstances and attitudes may prevent many coloured people from achieving professional or managerial status, with their attendant mental stresses. Lower social status did not protect patients in the Aberdeen survey.

Although this book is written about Crohn's disease, it does not rank among the top ten most common diseases in any community. Almy and Sherlock (1966) have calculated that with a prevalence rate of 20 per 100,000 the probability of familial occurrence due to chance alone is of the order of 1 in 25 million. If this calculation is correct, then there have been far too many familial examples reported to be accounted for by chance. Family must be important, but whether it is the genetic or the environmental aspect is uncertain. Both probably play some part. Husband and wife usually live longer together than parent and child, but Crohn's disease has not been recorded in husband and wife. From this point of view the genetic factor seems more important than the environmental one. The probability of occurrence by chance of concordance in monozygotic twins is 1 in over 6 billion, but 5 examples have been described (Hislop and Grant, 1969). Furthermore, Crohn's disease not infrequently is associated with other genetically determined conditions such as ankylosing spondylitis. Nevertheless, environment may be the reason for the Crohn's disease being observed more often in coloured Americans than in the inhabitants of central Africa, and for its rising incidence in the Bantu in Johannesburg (Girauld *et al.*, 1969).

The relationship between Crohn's disease and profession of the Jewish faith is difficult to unravel. The more recent experience at Mount Sinai Hospital throws doubt on whether there is any relationship. If one exists it is clearly not due to religion and theological concepts. It could be the result of numerous migrations over countless centuries, with intermarriage thereafter—Jews are not ethnically homogeneous. Special dietary regimes or respected cultural traditions such as methods of rearing a family may play a part, or it could be an interaction between any or all of these, between the macrocosm and the person's microcosm.

Industrialization may be responsible for Crohn's disease being commoner in Leeds and Baltimore than elsewhere. No large series have been reported from heavy industrial areas such as the Ruhr or northern Italy. There is a significant excess of patients with Crohn's disease in Aberdeen compared to the surrounding countryside, but Aberdeen is not industrialized. It is a relatively small city, most of whose citizens have close connections with the people in the rural districts.

Finally, it is probably true that the various preparatory factors and the precipitating agent (if there be one) must act and interact over long periods of time before finally giving rise to overt, clinical Crohn's disease. In the past attention has been focused largely on the patient's status at the time of onset. In the future it may be necessary to probe further back in time, which will be more difficult. Memory of events that happened 20 or 30 years ago is often unreliable. Adult patients may understandably resent being asked whether they were breast-fed and how they reacted to it! However, certain basic data such as place of birth and father's occupation could be obtained in a prospective study and, matched with suitable controls, might well prove valuable.

References

Acheson, E. D. (1960), *Gut*, **1**, 291.
Aktan, H. (1970), Personal communication.
Almy, T. P. and Sherlock, P. (1966), *Gastroenterology*, **51**, 757.
Anderson, J. G. D., Singer, H. C. and Kirsner, J. B. (1969), *Gastroenterology*, **56**, 1135.
Armitage, G. and Wilson, M. (1950), *Brit. J. Surg.*, **38**, 182.
Baird, D. A. (1970), Personal communication.
Baker, L. W. (1970), Personal communication.
Brom, B., Banks, S., Marks, I. N., Barbezat, G. O. and Raynham, B. (1968), *S. Afr. med. J.*, **42**, 1099.
Chacon, A. C. E. (1966), *Rev. Cuba Cir.*, **5**, 221.
Colcock, B. P. and Vansant, J. H. (1960), *Lahey Clin. Bull.*, **12**, 53.
Crohn, B. B. and Yarnis, H. (1958), *Regional Ileitis*, 2nd edition. New York: Grune and Stratton.
Cumming-Smith, C. (1970), Personal communication.
Daffner, J. E. and Brown, C. H. (1958), *Ann. Int. Med.*, **49**, 580.
De Beaux, J. (1970), Personal communication.
De Dombal, F. T. (1970), *Proc. Roy. Soc. Med.*, in press.
Edwards, H. C. (1964), *J. Roy. Coll. Surg. Edin.*, **9**, 115.
Edwards, H. C. (1969), *Ann. Roy. Coll. Surg. Eng.*, **44**, 121.
Evans, J. G. and Acheson, E. D. (1965), *Gut*, **6**, 311.
Ferrara, L. and Balbo, G. (1966), *Minerva Chir.*, **21**, 737.
Fielding, J. F. (1970a), *An Enquiry into Certain Aspects of Regional Enteritis*, M.D Thesis. National University of Ireland (Cork).
Fielding, J. F. (1970b), *Lancet*, **2**, 424.
Fone, D. J. (1966), *Med. J. Austral.*, **1**, 865.
Gentry, J. T., Nitowsky, H. M. and Michael, M. (1955), *J. Clin. Investig.*, **34**, 1839.
Gibson, J. B. (1970), Personal communication.
Gilbert, J. A. L. and Santor, V. E. (1964), *Canad. med. Ass. J.*, **91**, 23.
Girauld, R. M. A., Luke, I. and Schamaman, A. (1969), *S. Afr. med. J.*, **43**, 610.
Gjone, E., Orning, O. M. and Myren, J. (1966), *Gut*, **7**, 372.
Gjone, E. (1970), Personal communication.
Gupta, R. S., Chatterjee, A. K., Roy, R. and Ghosh, B. N. (1962), *Ind. J. Surg.*, **24**, 797.
Hall, G., Naish, P., Sharma, O. P., Doe, W. and James, D. G. (1969), *Postgrad. med. J.*, **45**, 241.
Harrison, F. S. V. (1970), *Burma*, p. 245. London: Ernest Benn.
Hislop, I. G. and Grant, A. K. (1969), *Gut*, **10**, 995.
Ishikura, H., Hayasaka, H. and Kikuchi, Y. (1967), *Sapporo. med. J.*, **32**, 183.
Jinch, H., Rojas, E. and Castro, R. (1967), *Gac. Med. Mex.*, **97**, 681.

Jonasson, H. (1970), Personal communication.
Kibaya, A. K. (1946), *E. Afr. Med. J.*, **23**, 317.
Kirsner, J. B. and Spencer, J. A. (1963), *Ann. Int. Med.*, **59**, 133.
Kubicki, S. (1964), *Pol. Tyg. Lek.*, **19**, 2011.
Kyle, J. (1971), *Gastroenterology*, **61**, 826.
Kyle, J., Adesola, A. O., Tinckler, L. F. and de Beaux, J. (1967), *Scand. J. Gastroent.*, **2**, 77.
Kyle, J. and Blair, D. W. (1965), *Brit. J. Surg.*, **52**, 215.
Lennard-Jones, J. E. (1968), *Proc. Roy. Soc. Med.*, **61**, 81.
Lewisohn, R. (1938), *Surg. Gynec. Obstet.*, **66**, 215.
McGovern, V. J. and Goulston, S. J. M. (1968), *Gut*, **9**, 164.
Maratka, Z. (1968), *Digestion*, **1**, 251.
Martinez, G. M. (1968), *Arch. Col. Med. El Salvador*, **21**, 284.
Mendeloff, A. I., Monk, M., Siegel, C. I. and Lilienfeld, A. (1966), *Gastroenterology*, **51**, 748.
Monk, M., Mendeloff, A. I., Siegel, C. I. and Lilienfeld, A. (1969), *Gastroenterology*, **56**, 847.
Monk, M., Mendeloff. A. I., Siegel, C. I. and Lilienfeld, A. (1970), *J. Chr. Dis.*, **22**, 565.
Morl, F. K. (1966), *Beitr. Klin. Chir.*, **213**, 285.
Norlen, B. J., Krause, U. and Bergman, L. (1970), *Scand. J. Gastroent.*, **5**, 385.
Ratzloff, N. and Jacobs, W. H. (1970), *Amer. J. Gastroent.*, **53**, 252.
Rozen, P. (1970), Personal communication.
Ruble, P. E., Meyers, S. G. and Ashley, L. B. (1957), *Harper Hosp. Bull.*, **15**, 142.
Saidi, F. (1970). Personal communication.
Sharma. A. K. (1966), Personal communication.
Vantrappen, G., Lens, E., Vandenbroucke, J., Bodart, P. and Dive, C. (1966), *Arch. Franc. Mal. Appar. Digest.*, **55**, 1129.
Van Patter, W. N., Bargen, J. A., Dockerty, M. B., Feldman, W. H., Mayo, C. W. and Waugh, J. M. (1954), *Gastroenterology*, **16**, 25.
Warthin, T. A. (1968), *Trans. Amer. Clin. Climat. Ass.*, **80**, 116.
Wigley, R. D. and Maclaurin, B. P. (1962), *Brit. med. J.*, **2**, 228.
Wright, J. T. (1970), *Proc. 4th World Congress of Gastroenterology*, Copenhagen.
Yamase, K., Masuda, K., Shimada, S. and Yamada, Y. (1967), *Int. Surg.*, **47**, 497.
Yovanovich, M. B. Y. (1961), *Arch. Mal. Appar. Dig.*, **50**, 1062.

Chapter III
Aetiology

No single factor has been identified which alone can produce chronic Crohn's disease. It may be a disease with a multi-factorial pathogenesis. Indeed it is not certain that it is a single pathological entity (Chess *et al.*, 1950). It may only be a clinical syndrome produced by a variety of agents, the intestine having a limited range of cellular response to different forms of insult and injury. If this latter suggestion is correct, it is surprising that no histological appearance identical to that of Crohn's disease has been produced in various experiments. Even allowing for the fact that the experiments have been conducted in other species, very few of the resulting granulomas closely resembled those of Crohn's disease. The lack of similarity must have dissuaded other workers from repeating the experiments. One of the curious features of attempts to produce Crohn's disease is that most of the results remain uncorroborated.

In spite of the lack of success during nearly four decades, new aetiological theories are put forward at intervals, and new experiments are devised. It is likely to be very difficult to produce a chronic disease in animals which will last for a long period of time like the human counterpart. The few granulomatous conditions that develop spontaneously in animals only last for a short time and are not really comparable to chronic Crohn's disease.

Granulomatous Disease of the Intestine in Animals
In Scandinavia a transmural type of inflammation is seen in the lower ileum of pigs (Emsbo, 1951); the incidence is very much greater than that of Crohn's disease in humans (Adsersen, 1931). The porcine disease occurs in two age periods—in piglets a few weeks old, and in mature pigs ready for slaughter. In the piglets the condition appears to be an infection, runs a rapid course and the animals mostly die from perforation of the ileum. This condition resembles enteritis necroticans of humans (Smith, 1969) rather than Crohn's disease. Mature pigs that are otherwise healthy are sometimes found to have marked thickening of the muscle in the terminal ileum. There is little or no ulceration of the mucosa. Changes in the muscularis propria are slight or absent in Crohn's disease.

Strande *et al.* (1954) described a granulomatous process in the ileal wall of two Cocker spaniel dogs that became ill with diarrhoea and vomiting. The lesions seem to have been mainly in the colon where there was "discontinuous pathology". The thickened bowel wall showed submucous oedema, and some granulomas were present both there and in the liver. Epithelioid cells were not prominent, the few giant cells noted were of foreign-body rather than Langhans type, and there was marked tissue eosinophilia although no parasites were detected. Nevertheless, these two Cocker spaniels had a disease which more closely resembled Crohn's disease than did any of the other animal conditions that have been described. Boxer dogs occasionally develop a colitis (Kennedy and Cello, 1966), but the abnormality is confined to the mucosa and submucosa; large macrophages similar to those seen in Johnne's disease of cattle are present.

Theories on the Aetiology of Crohn's Disease

The theories that have been advanced can be considered under 10 main headings. In the years immediately after the first description of the disease attention was focused on the possibility of lymphatic obstruction, ingested materials, or of the classical types of bacteria being responsible. Virus studies came later. The relationship between Crohn's disease, sarcoidosis and tuberculosis has been in dispute for many years. As larger series of patients accumulated it was recognized that a familial factor might be operative and a small number of cases followed severe abdominal trauma. The possibility that Crohn's disease might have a psychosomatic basis has been considered. An allergic or hypersensitivity cause for Crohn's disease has often been suspected; the damage sustained by the intestine may be the result of an immunopathological phenomenon. In recent years attention has been directed largely towards filter-passing particles and immunological reactions, but none of the factors mentioned above has been completely excluded. Several of them almost certainly play a preparatory or potentiating role in at least some of the patients who clinically have Crohn's disease.

1. Lymphatic Obstruction

Enlargement of regional lymph nodes and oedema of the submucosa, visible to the naked eye, are two of the earliest features of Crohn's disease; mucosal ulceration may be a secondary change. Obstruction to the flow of lymph from the intestine might produce the appearances observed. Reichert and Mathes (1936) tried sclerosing the lymphatics in dogs by injecting them directly with sclerosants such as bismuth oxychloride, silica, rose aniline dye and sodium morrhuate. In addition some animals were given an intravenous infusion of a suspension of *Escherichia Coli* some hours beforehand. The result was that most dogs developed chronic lymphoedema of the bowel wall; initially some acute inflammatory cells were present, to be replaced later by a few round cells. The lymph nodes became enlarged and the lymphatics were dilated. There was marked thickening of the muscle coat, but the mucosa remained intact and the animals seemed well. It is difficult to obtain ulceration by lymphatic blockage (Sinaiko *et al.*, 1946).

Bockus and Lee (1935) had suggested that there might be a lymphangitis, presumably of bacterial origin. Proliferating endothelial cells and lymphoid aggregates have also been blamed for obstructing the lymphatics. Bockus and Lee developed their theory by suggesting that infection spread from the lymphatics to the blood vessels, causing local devitalization of the intestinal wall. However, Bell (1934) had been unable to produce Crohn's disease in animals by interfering with the mesenteric blood supply.

A recent study (Kalima and Collan, 1970) on experimental lymphatic obstruction in rats has provided information on the state of the lymphatics in the villus in early and late obstruction. After a few days the endothelial lining cells simply looked stretched, and oedema fluid had separated the collagen fibres. When animals were sacrificed after a month there was transmural inflammation (in one rat a fistula had formed). Polymorphonuclear leucocytes, lymphocytes and plasma cells were present and some macrophages contained phagocytosed material. The endothelial cells of the lymphatics also had fat deposits, pinocytosis vacuoles and fibrillary changes in the cytoplasm. The muscle layer was clearly thickened but there were no granulomas. The changes were more like those of congenital intestinal lymphangiectasis (Dobbins, 1966) than Crohn's disease.

It remains uncertain whether the dilatation of lymphatics and intestinal oedema observed in Crohn's disease are the result of excessive outpouring of interstitial fluid, paralysis of and stasis within the lymphatics or to their obstruction either by masses of hyperplastic cells in wall or nodes, or else by lymphangitis and endothelial proliferation.

2. Ingested Foreign Material

The rising incidence of Crohn's disease suggests that some factor in the modern way of living might be of aetiological significance. New methods of processing food, additives to and contaminants of various foodstuffs and dental hygiene preparations have all been suspected. Compounds of aluminium, barium, molybdenum and titanium and the elements beryllium and zirconium can cause granuloma-formation in the tissue. Asbestos, cholesterol and quartz particles produce a similar effect; distortion of their asymmetrically arranged atoms generates small charges of piezoelectricity, which may act as a local irritant. Chess *et al.* (1950) tried instilling sand and talc into Thierry loops of ileum in dogs. After a time considerable lymphoid hyperplasia was obtained, with granulomas containing giant cells in the ileal wall; the regional nodes were hyperplastic and some adhesions formed. The granulomas were composed of chronic inflammatory cells rather than the epithelioid cells of Crohn's disease and the giant cells were of foreign-body type. Feeding dogs sand or talc produced a friable, haemorrhagic mucosa; the haemorrhagic tendency could be exaggerated by giving an intravenous injection of an *Escherichia Coli* suspension. Silica granulomas were noted in the liver.

There are several thousand chemical substances, natural or synthetic, added to the food that is consumed in Western countries (Carstensen and Poulsen, 1971). Some such as iron and vitamins are beneficial; others such as thickeners are probably inert. However, many preservatives, anti-oxidants, dyes, flavours and maturing agents are more potent and their toxic potential in man has not been fully evaluated. Singly or acting synergistically they might have deleterious effects either directly on the intestine, on its secretions or on the normal bacterial flora. Carrageenan, a sulphated polysaccharide, extracted from seaweed, when fed to small rodents, can produce a condition like ulcerative colitis (Marcus and Watt, 1969). Strenuous efforts have been made during the past decade to eliminate or greatly reduce the concentration of contaminants in foodstuffs, particularly pesticides and toxins from fungi.

Partial or abnormal breakdown of food constituents during digestion could challenge the intestinal mucosa and absorptive mechanisms with products that they were unable to deal with. There is little evidence of phagocytosis and none of abnormal fatty acids in the inner layers of the intestinal wall in patients with Crohn's disease. There do not appear to be any major defects or deficiencies of small intestinal enzymes that might permit abnormal breakdown products of food to be present in the wall. Some impairment in the handling of lactose (Chalfin and Holt, 1967) may be the result rather than the cause of the disease. This relationship may also be true of some of the other observations mentioned later in this chapter.

While an unusual reaction to some ingested material is a remote possibility, at the present time there is no suggestive, let alone convincing evidence, that any such material is the cause of Crohn's disease.

3. Bacterial Infection
During the 7 years before the outbreak of the Second World War the possible role of numerous classical types of bacteria in the aetiology of Crohn's disease was studied by various workers. Felsen (1936) suggested that a proportion of cases followed bacillary dysentery. Among the men in the Aberdeen series of patients there were 6 who had had dysentery (bacillary or amoebic) while serving in the Armed Forces in Africa or Asia. Many years had elapsed before they started to get symptoms of Crohn's disease; culture of their stools revealed no pathogens and amoeba could not be demonstrated. There is unlikely to be any cause and effect relationship between dysentery and Crohn's disease. Only one out of the 400 patients who had typhoid fever in Aberdeen in 1964 is

known to have developed Crohn's disease two years later; this could have happened by chance.

Most other types of easily grown bacteria, for example streptococci, have also been exonerated. It must be remembered that many of the organisms in the lower small intestine and colon are anaerobic and can only be studied when special collection and culture techniques are employed. A detailed investigation of intestinal flora is a time-consuming exercise, requiring a great many sub-cultures. In two patients with Crohn's disease, Gorbach and Tabaqchali (1969) noted excessive growth of bacteroides in the area of stasis above the stenosed distal ileum. The 6 patients studied by Drasar and Shiner (1969) had had resections and so presumably had no stasis; nevertheless they too had a noticeable growth of bacteroides as well as of yeasts, enterobacteria, fusobacteria and bifidobacteria from intestinal samples.

Bacteria are not numerous on histological sections of diseased ileum. The surface distribution of organisms is not even; there are clusters or plaques of bacteria (Tabaqchali, 1970) and the effect they may have on adjacent mucosa obviously might be important. It is not certain if secretory immunoglobulins (IgA) are able to regulate the flora of the intestinal tract. There are plenty of plasma cells containing IgA in the jejunal wall in Crohn's disease (Soltoft, 1969). The faecal count of coliforms may rise and fall with relapses and remissions respectively. However, Crohn's disease is probably not caused by direct bacterial invasion of the mucosa and deeper layers of the ileum. Toxins liberated in the lumen might play some part in aetiology. Prohaska (1966) claimed that by injecting staphylococcal exotoxin into the lumen of the ileum he could produce chronic enteritis (with skip areas) in experimental animals.

Alternatively, bacteria might act by interfering with normal absorptive and catabolic processes within the bowel. They are able to hydrolyse bile acid conjugates (Drasar and Shiner, 1969; Aries *et al.*, 1969), and may participate in the breakdown of steroids and cholesterol. The bile salt pattern in thoracic duct lymph was normal in 5 patients, although they had higher levels of cholesterol than normal individuals (Ghoos and Vantrappen, 1970). Some bacteria can manufacture essential food factors, for example vitamin K and folic acid; other bacteria may cannabalize certain food constituents and alter fat absorption. These perhaps minor alterations in small bowel function brought about by bacterial activity may in part account for some of the features of Crohn's disease; it is improbable that they are a major factor in causation.

The investigation of anaerobic bacteria and of wall-deficient types and phage-infected mycobacteria is only just beginning. The latter are almost impossible to demonstrate and culture by currently available techniques. Morganroth and Watson (1970) failed to demonstrate sensitivity to atypical mycobacterial antigens in patients with Crohn's disease.

Mesenteric adenitis and terminal ileitis can result from infection with *Yersinia Pseudotuberculosis*, which is normally a pathogen in rodents and birds (Winblad *et al.*, 1966). In the past such human cases may have been labelled as acute Crohn's disease, but clearly this was erroneous. It is not certain whether *Yersinia Pseudotuberculosis* is the same organism as Russian workers (Arapov *et al.*, 1971) claim to have isolated in 32 out of 76 cases of Crohn's disease; they describe it as a pseudo-tuberculous microbe but do not positively identify it.

Particular attention has been directed towards the possible role that the tubercle bacillus and other mycobacteria may play in the aetiology of Crohn's disease. The lesions produced in cattle by *M. Johneii* under the microscope do not closely resemble those seen in Crohn's disease. The incidence of the latter disease has slowly increased during the past three decades which have witnessed a dramatic fall in the incidence of tuberculosis in Europe and elsewhere. When acid- and alcohol-fast bacilli or caseation are demonstrated in granulomatous lesions in the wall of the intestine, the case is considered tuberculous. Goldie (1968) suggested that Crohn's disease might be caused by some as yet unidenti-fied mycobacterium, and produced dermatological and pharmacological analogies in support of his argument. An alternative explanation was put forward by Fielding (1970). His theory was that when resistance was low, exposure to *Mycobacterium tuberculosis* resulted in clinical tuberculosis; when resistance was moderate, sarcoidosis might result, while with even high resistance the disease would be well localized, the mycobacteria would be killed and only Crohn's granulomatous lesion remain. Among patients being diagnosed as having Crohn's disease today it is rare to encounter one who has previously had tuberculosis. A few patients with advanced and recurrent Crohn's disease became malnourished, and it is not surprising that one or two of these unlucky patients later develop pulmonary tuberculosis. This does not establish a cause and effect relationship between the tubercle bacillus and Crohn's disease.

Although the intact *M. tuberculosis* does not cause Crohn's disease, the possibility remains that some antigenic breakdown product may be implicated. Originally it was believed that the Mantoux tuberculin skin test was mostly negative in Crohn's disease, particularly when discrete granulomas were present (Williams, 1965). However, when purified tuberculin of proven potency is used, a positive skin reaction can usually be obtained (Fletcher and Hinton, 1967). The attenuated organism used in B.C.G. vaccination has been both incriminated in the causation (Campbell and Shaw, 1966) and credited with producing marked improvement in Crohn's disease (Geffroy *et al.*, 1970). The patient's immunological status at the time of exposure to the foreign protein may in part account for these bizarre findings which admittedly might have occurred by chance.

4. Viruses

During the past 15 years techniques for culturing viruses and for identifying antibodies have developed considerably. In Aberdeen 35 patients with Crohn's disease were studied by Dr T. Bell to see if viruses were responsible for their condition. Specimens of sera were obtained from all the patients. They were tested for the presence of adenovirus group antibody by complement fixation tests and for the six group B Coxsackie viruses by neutralization tests. When any antibody was demonstrated the exact titre was determined by serial doubling dilutions up to 1 in 320. Repeat tests were carried out in half the patients for up to one year. Table 1 shows the antibody results in the patients compared

Table 1

Viral antibody titres in a series of 35 patients with Crohn's disease and in 108 normal controls (expressed as percentage of each series)

(a) *Antibody Titres to Adenovirus*

	Titre = less than 1:4	Titre = 1:32 or more
Crohn's disease	55	10
Controls	50	12

(b) *Antibody Titres to Coxsackie Group B*

	Titre = 1:5 or less						Titre = 1:320 or more					
-----------------	B_1	B_2	B_3	B_4	B_5	B_6	B_1	B_2	B_3	B_4	B_5	B_6
Virus type												
Crohn's disease	87	28	86	80	100	100	0	12	0	0	0	0
Controls	70	33	65	42	90	94	2	12	2	3	1	0

with those in 108 normal members of the population at the time (1961–1963). There is no significant difference between the test and the control groups (Kyle *et al*, 1963.)

Pieces of diseased ileum from 10 patients and lymph nodes from 6 were cultured. Two culture techniques were employed, explanting small fragments at 34°C in plasma clot, and by suspension cultures incubated at 37°C in roller tubes. Cultures on human amnion, embryo kidney and Hela cells were continued for 5 weeks. No viruses were grown from any of the specimens in spite of the proved efficacy of the methods that were used. Schneierson *et al.* (1962) had obtained similar negative results at the Mount Sinai Hospital, New York.

In 1963 Tomenius *et al.* reported that they had obtained positive Frei tests in 7 patients with Crohn's disease. The antigen had been prepared from the brains of mice infected with the virus of lymphogranuloma venereum. Tests in control subjects were negative, and the Swedish workers felt it was logical to regard a virus as a probable agent capable of producing Crohn's disease. The author performed Frei tests on 7 patients with proven Crohn's disease of colon and rectum and on 3 patients with the ileal form of the disease. All were negative. Unfortunately no patient with lymphogranuloma was available in the region, so that the potency of the material used could not be verified. No other reports of positive Frei tests have appeared. Later Tomenius (1968) remarked that Crohn's disease sometimes became manifest after an attack of influenza or tonsillitis. He suggested that infection of the lymphoid tissue of the upper respiratory tract and of the gut might be important. These types of infection are common and by chance some cases of Crohn's disease could develop a few weeks or months after any of them. The cytomegalovirus has not been studied in Crohn's disease.

Considerable interest has been aroused by the paper of Mitchell and Rees (1970) on "an agent transmissible from Crohn's disease tissue". They made homogenates from fresh mesenteric nodes and ileal wall of a patient with proven Crohn's disease, using 1 per cent bovine albumin. These were injected into the footpads of normal and of prepared immunologically-deficient mice. For a control series, a homogenate was prepared from normal para-aortic or inguinal lymph nodes. In addition, all homogenates were injected into guinea-pigs and cultured on Lowenstein medium. Biopsies were taken from the footpads at intervals of from 26 to 500 days. In a high portion of the animals that had received Crohn's disease homogenate typical epithelioid cell-granulomas, with occasional Langhans giant cells, slowly developed. The immunological state of the animal did not seem to make much difference. Kveim tests were performed on the ears of the test group mice; 6 out of 17 gave positive results on histological examination. Only 1 out of 58 mice given non-Crohn's lymph node homogenate showed a transient granulomatous response in its footpad; none showed a positive Kveim reaction. No mycobacterium was cultured from any of the homogenates.

Mitchell and Rees (1970) have not called their "transmissible agent" a virus. They have not demonstrated any mycobacterium, so that the assumption may be made that the particle is virus-size or smaller. However, at the present time the nature of the particle in their unfiltered homogenate of Crohn's tissue is not known. The same workers had reported in 1969 that there was a transmissible agent in sarcoidosis. Earlier, Sanders (1964) failed to produce a reaction by injecting a Crohn's lymph node homogenate intradermally in 9 patients with Crohn's disease.

5. Sarcoidosis

The relationship, if any, between Crohn's disease and sarcoidosis is baffling. Histologically the typical granulomas of both conditions look very similar (Phear, 1958; Williams, 1965), although Crohn's disease embraces a wider spectrum of cellular patterns. Skin, joint and eye complications of comparable types may appear in both diseases. In spite of these apparent similarities, the differences are more numerous and probably more important. The epidemiology of sarcoidosis does not resemble that of Crohn's disease (page 13). In America, sarcoidosis is relatively more common in the south-east states, in females, and in the coloured population; the prevalence of Crohn's disease is greatest among northern, white males. Around London many sufferers from sarcoid are of Irish descent. The principal lesion in sarcoidosis is in the lungs and most cases resolve spontaneously. A very few patients may show a transient sarcoid reaction in the gastric mucosa, but the lower small intestine is not affected. By contrast, Crohn's disease shows no tendency to cure itself and the distal ileum is the part most frequently involved. So far as is known no patients who have had sarcoidosis have later developed Crohn's disease, or *vice versa*.

Kveim's intradermal test originally was considered specific for sarcoidosis (Williams, 1965). On simple inspection of injected sites in patients with Crohn's disease the reaction seemed to be negative. However, Mitchell *et al.* (1969) using validated sarcoid antigen, and performing skin biopsies 28 to 42 days after injection, have been able to show that a positive granulomatous reaction occurs in 50 per cent of Crohn's patients; 90 per cent of patients with sarcoidosis react. The material which Mitchell used for the Kveim test was not necessarily identical with the "transmissible agent" contained in the homogenate, although it may have been a part of or associated with the latter. A Kveim suspension is capable of inhibiting the migration of leucocytes in 2 out of 3 patients with Crohn's disease (Willoughby and Mitchell, 1971). This observation suggests cross-reactivity or a possible aetiological link between sarcoidosis and Crohn's disease.

6. Heredity

The occasional appearance of Crohn's disease or ulcerative colitis in more than one member of a family has already been referred to (page 16). Among the families of the 166 Aberdeen patients with Crohn's disease there was one where the mother of the patient had Crohn's disease and three families in which a first degree relative had ulcerative colitis. Thus there was a familial incidence of inflammatory bowel disease in almost 3 per cent of families. Conversely no familial influence was apparent in 97 per cent of cases. Unless all first degree relatives of a patient are themselves directly questioned a few familial examples may be missed and the familial influence seem falsely low.

The association between Crohn's disease and other conditions which show a familial tendency such as ankylosing spondylitis (McBride *et al.*, 1963) and eczema (Hammer *et al.*, 1967) strengthens the belief that inheritance may sometimes be of importance. The inherited, sex-linked deficiency of glucose-6-phosphate enzyme in red blood cells was at one time thought to be commoner in patients with Crohn's disease (Sheehan *et al.*, 1967), but other workers (Katsaros and Truelove, 1969) found no evidence of such an association. Nevertheless in some patients an inherited factor may prepare the way for Crohn's disease (or ulcerative colitis) to develop in later life.

7. Trauma

More than thirty years ago workers at the Mayo Clinic reported that Crohn's disease could follow direct external injury to the abdomen (Morlock *et al.*, 1939). Trauma to the intestine has been mentioned by virtually everyone who since then has written about the possible cause of Crohn's disease. Unfortunately they have added little fresh information and the concept is in some danger of becoming hallowed by repetition rather than by the frequency of its occurrence. Edwards (1969) had 13 patients out of a series of over 300 who blamed abdominal trauma for causing their disease. This incidence of 4 per cent is the highest that has been recorded, but Edwards advises caution in accepting the patients' explanation. The pain of injury may only have drawn their attention to intestinal disease that was already slowly and silently appearing. In the Aberdeen series there was only one patient in whom the timing of events gave grounds for believing that a severe crush injury of the abdomen might have been responsible for Crohn's disease found at laparotomy some weeks later.

Trauma might act by releasing into the circulation antigenic material not normally present there. It might also damage the blood supply. Following transient strangulation of colon in an umbilical hernia, a patient developed obstructive signs necessitating operation a few days later. At laparotomy, a 15 cm segment of transverse colon was markedly thickened, with a matt serosal surface. The gross appearances looked like Crohn's disease, but the findings on histological examination bore no resemblance to those of the granulomatous condition. No case is known where vascular embarrassment has progressed to chronic, relapsing Crohn's disease.

8. Diverticula

Diverticula of the jejunum were noted in 7 out of the 166 patients. In 3 patients they may have been pseudo-diverticula, the result of stenotic lesions immediately beyond them. In the remaining patients the diverticula were multiple and separated by a considerable length of normal looking intestine from the area of Crohn's disease in the lower ileum. The significance of this finding is not clear. Jejunal diverticula are said to be present in about 1·25 per cent of adults coming to autopsy (Christensen, 1969). It must be remembered that Crohn's disease constitutes one of the few reasons for examining the intestine from end to end, looking for skip lesions. Such a careful search might give a false impression that the incidence of other intestinal lesions was abnormally high. Bianco (1966) and Debray (1969) have also described Crohn's disease in association with upper small intestinal diverticula. Aubrey (1970) reviewed 66 patients in whom a Meckel's diverticulum had been found at emergency laparotomy. Five had Crohn's disease and 30 had acute appendicitis; this is a ratio of 1 : 6 although acute appendicitis is several hundred times more common than any acute presentation of Crohn's disease. Schmidt *et al.* (1968) have given a useful description of how to differentiate between Crohn's disease and diverticulitis of the colon. Both diseases may present in the older age groups, and they may coexist. The possibility that mural damage caused by diverticulitis initiates a sequence of events that finally manifests itself as colonic Crohn's disease has not been eliminated. Clark (1969) has described microdiverticula, less than 1 mm in diameter, in both ileum and colon. His suggestion is that foreign material, possibly of a lipid nature, entering and irritating these microdiverticula, may provoke a granulomatous response.

9. Psychological Factors

There is no unequivocal evidence that psychological factors are responsible for Crohn's disease. It is becoming increasingly difficult for an ordinary surgeon to understand the terminology and tests used by psychiatrists. It is relatively simple for him to decide whether the behaviour and attitude of the patients with Crohn's disease who attend his clinic differ noticeably from those of other patients with abdominal complaints. In the author's opinion they do not. Bockus (1945) thought his Crohn's patients were emotional, sensitive and some were severely psychoneurotic. Wells (1949) remarked on the fortitude shown by these patients (and those with ulcerative colitis) in spite of years of ill health. Crockett (1952) and Whybrow *et al.* (1968) thought the patients were unusually liable to depressive swings, but Goldberg (1970) found no proof of this among 23 patients with Crohn's disease. Children with Crohn's disease are said to be depressed at times (Reinhart and Succop, 1968). Who would blame them? As Avery Jones and Gummer (1960) have remarked, the influence may be as much somatopsychic as psychosomatic. Feldman *et al.* (1967) were unable to detect any particular personality characteristic predisposing to the disease. After analysing the personality differences between patients with all types of inflammatory bowel disease and their normal siblings, McMahon *et al.* (1971) concluded that the patients were more conscientious and conforming, the unaffected siblings more rebellious and independent. Clinicians responsible for long-term care can only be thankful that their patients are not particularly rebellious!

Nine per cent of Edward's (1969) King's College Hospital patients needed psychiatric treatment at some time compared to 5 per cent among the 212 controls. However, the latter group have not had to endure chronic illness; repeated relapses must give rise to great disappointment as well as to deterioration in the unfortunate patient's general health. Among the Aberdeen patients, 7 per cent had received psychiatric treatment. Goldberg (1970) did not consider that malnutrition or specific deficiencies were related to psychiatric illness, but most of the Aberdeen patients with psychiatric trouble did have severe, protracted Crohn's disease.

It is just possible that stressful events in life may precipitate a relapse. There is some evidence that stress may interfere with immunological responses (Solomons, 1969).

10. Immunopathology

Crohn's disease may recur from 15 to 20 years after apparently success-ful ileal resection. This late type of recurrence is a major disappointment to both patient and surgeon. Any theory about the aetiology of Crohn's disease must be capable of explaining it. Some micro-organisms, such as the mycobacteria, can remain dormant for many years. The few patients in Britain who today show evidence of tuberculosis probably inhaled or ingested the mycobacteria 25–50 years ago. Leprosy can be a very chronic disease (Golde, 1967). It is not known with certainty for how long a virus may remain active; the herpes virus can probably lie dormant within a cell for years. Another possibility is that an immuno-pathological process is involved. "Immunological memory" is believed to be very long and consequently an abnormality of the immune response might account for the protracted life history of Crohn's disease.

Immunological reactions are of two types—

(1) Immediate hypersensitivity, probably the result of circulating humoral antibodies that have been formed in lymph nodes and other peripheral parts of the lymphoid system. The antibodies are immuno-globins subdivided into various classes. The macroglobulin IgM is the first antibody to be formed after an antigenic challenge, to be followed later by IgG. When they react with antigen complement becomes activated and attacks the offending bacteria or surrounding cells, causing tissue damage. IgE is known as the reaginic antibody. The IgA fraction appears in the lumen of the gut and does not require the pre-sence of complement to be effective. It is not known whether the different types of gammaglobulins all come from one cell or from different clones of lymphoid cells, but probably a correct balance between them is necessary for normal health. Variations in their concentration in disease may be either the result or the cause of fluctuations in activity. The strength and timing of the antigenic challenge is probably relevant.

(2) Delayed hypersensitivity which is mediated by lymphocytes and is largely dependent on the central lymphoid tissue in the thymus. Lymphocytes that have passed through the thymus appear to have antigen receptor groups similar to antibody incorporated in their cell membrane. They do not need complement to be present in order to attack antigen-containing structures.

The ileo-caecal region of the intestine is the part most commonly attacked by Crohn's disease. It contains a large amount of lymphoid tissue, for example in Peyer's patches, but whether this should be regarded as central or peripheral lymphoid tissue is not certain; the latter is more probable. However, it is clear that this part of the intestine could act as a powerful production organ in the immunological system as well as being a potential target for an immunological reaction.

While there is no single piece of evidence that constitutes conclusive proof that Crohn's disease is the result of altered reactivity of the immune mechanism of the body, there are a number of clinical and experimental observations which, when considered together, strongly suggest that this is in fact the case.

Clinical Observations

Crohn's disease runs a chronic relapsing course, not unlike that of rheumatoid arthritis which has an immunopathological basis. Various types of skin lesion may appear in unpredictable fashion in a patient with Crohn's disease. Among the most striking is erythema nodosum, which is believed to be caused by a hypersensitivity reaction with vasculitis. In earlier life the patient may have had eczema. Iritis and uveitis in the eye and flitting arthritis in major joints are occasional features of Crohn's disease, and all are possibly caused by altered reactivity. Milk proteins cause an immune response in a proportion of patients with ulcerative colitis, but not in Crohn's disease (Taylor *et al.*, 1964). The Kveim test has already been discussed (page 34). While there is now grave doubt about its specificity, the granulomatous reaction which it provokes in the skin is strongly suggestive of an immunopathological reaction.

Deficient or defective immunological response could be damaging to the patient. Some years ago when uncontrolled Mantoux skin tests appeared to indicate that this test was frequently negative in patients with Crohn's disease it was postulated that these patients exhibited anergy or failure to mount a delayed hypersensitivity (cell-mediated) response. Carefully controlled Mantoux testing was then performed by Fletcher and Hinton (1967) who demonstrated quite clearly that the majority of patients did react to potent tuberculin. Binder *et al.* (1966) showed that a good delayed hypersensitivity response to three different antigens could be obtained. There may be some impairment of the reaction to the chemical dinitrochlorobenzene (Jones *et al.*, 1969). However, this is an artificial challenge, the result has not been confirmed by others, and it might simply have been caused by the patient's general ill health (Lennard-Jones and Morson, 1969). Gross deficiencies of circulating immunoglobins are rare. With one type of hypogamma-globulinaemia there may be extensive ulceration of the jejunum and ileum (Corlin and Pops, 1971), but without the granulomatous thickening which is such a striking feature of Crohn's disease.

An immunopathological process might be reflected in the metabolism of the immunoglobulins. Estimation of these circulating antibodies is not easy. Results reported sometimes vary. Such variations may be due to the experience of, and the technique used at, any particular centre, as well as to the activity of the patient's disease. The serum level of IgG is said to be raised in 30 per cent of cases of Crohn's disease, and normal in the remainder (Bendixen *et al.*, 1968). The catabolic rate of IgG is greatly increased; some of the immunoglobulin may become fixed in the intestinal wall (Schofield *et al.*, 1968). The serum level of the macroglublin fraction IgM is mostly normal (Jensen *et al.*, 1970), but again the turnover is increased and is independent of the total protein loss through the intestine. Serum IgA levels are reported to be mostly within normal limits; IgA found in the lumen of the intestine has had a secretory piece added to it by the epithelial cells (Tomasi *et al.*, 1965). During an acute exacerbation of Crohn's disease there may be a transient rise in serum IgA, but in prolonged and unresponsive disease the IgA, IgG and IgM levels all tend to be lower than normal (Weeke and Jarnum, 1971).

Both corticosteroids and immunosuppressive drugs such as azathioprine modify immune reactions. They have been used in the treatment of Crohn's disease (Chap. VIII). They are capable of bringing about considerable improvement during an acute flare-up of symptoms, but their long-term effects are uncertain. Nevertheless, the initial therapeutic response does suggest that there is an underlying immunopathological process at work. The use of antibiotics in Crohn's disease has not proved to be very helpful. Broad-spectrum antibiotics can markedly affect the intestinal flora during the time they are being given. Obviously this could alter the antigenic challenge to the gut wall, if antigens contained in bacteria are important. Once antibiotics are stopped, any temporary improvement in symptoms is soon lost.

The granulomatous reaction seen in two-thirds of resected specimens of Crohn's disease is very suggestive of an immunopathological reaction. So-called epithelioid cells are usually grouped into discrete granulomas (page 55). These may be found in any part of the intestinal wall, but mostly in the submucous layer and in relation to lymphoid tissue. Langhan's giant cells are frequently present. In some patients the granulomatous reaction is more diffuse, or the transmural inflammation may be of less specific character. Although not always present, granulomas are one of the more valuable pieces of evidence implicating an immune reaction in the aetiology of Crohn's disease. It would be interesting to know the state of the thymus in the disease. Abnormalities might be expected during an immunopathological disease (Asherson, 1967), but in a primary immunological structure enlargement would not occur in response to an exogenous stimulus. Few patients die in the acute phase, so that opportunities for direct examination must be very rare. When death follows a prolonged period of malnutrition and sepsis the thymus is likely to have undergone involution.

Experimental Observations

Those antibodies that are referred to as auto-antibodies are a somewhat ill-defined group. It is unlikely that the unaltered protein of a patient, being truly "self", would provoke a defence reaction. Probably if a component of a human cell is to act as an effective antigen in that person, it must first be modified or altered in some subtle way, possibly by an extraneous agent, so that the immune system considers it to be "non-self" and reacts accordingly. In Aberdeen Dr I. Porteous tested the sera of 32 patients with Crohn's disease to see if he could detect the presence in them of anti-colonic antibodies that Broberger and Perlmann (1959) had found in children with ulcerative colitis. Using the immuno-fluorescent and double-diffusion in agar techniques he was unable to demonstrate any reaction against a preparation of human colonic cells. Marataka (1961) and Koffler *et al.* (1962) reported similar negative results. Eighteen Aberdeen patients had their sera tested for anti-nuclear, anti-thyroid and anti-gastric antibodies, but none were found; Harrison (1965), too, failed to demonstrate this group of antibodies in 42 patients with Crohn's disease.

Lymphocytes from patients with Crohn's disease are cytotoxic for preparations of colonic cells, but they are not toxic towards ileal cells. Their colonic cytotoxicity is soon lost after resection; it may be inhibited by an extract of *Escherichia coli* (Shorter *et al.*, 1970). Loss of the feedback mechanism may explain why resection should terminate the state of cytotoxicity in lymphocytes. *Escherichia coli* contains antigens similar to those in epithelial cells; these antigens might saturate receptor sites on sensitized lymphocytes. On exposure to colonic or faecal extract there appears to be a blast-cell transformation reaction in the lymphocytes of patients with Crohn's disease, as measured by their ability to take up labelled thymidine (Pinedo and Watson, 1971). Normal lymphocytes appear relatively inactive; the exact purpose of increased activity in Crohn's disease is not known, but it may well be concerned with an immunological role. Bendixen (1967) observed that mixed peripheral blood leucocytes from patients did not have their *in vitro* migration inhibited by colonic or jejuno-ileal homogenate. He interpreted this as possibly indicating an alteration in the delayed type of hypersensitivity. The ability of polymorphonuclear leucocytes to phagocytose bacteria in Crohn's disease merits investigation. Aluwihare (1971) has noticed bacteria deep to seemingly intact epithelium in patients; if they are doing any harm it may be of an immunological type rather than a direct toxic effect on the surface.

The "transmissible agent" of Mitchell and Rees (1970) produces a granulomatous reaction; the agent may be an antigen and is not necessarily a virus or micro-organism capable of reproduction. Slaney (1962) succeeded in producing granulomas in the intestinal wall of rabbits by sensitizing them to horse serum and later injecting horse serum into the subserosal layer of the wall. The lesions bore some resemblance to those of Crohn's disease, but it is not known how chronic they were, or if they were self-perpetuating.

These experimental observations are less convincing support for an immunological aetiology in Crohn's disease than are the clinical observations. Among the latter the histological appearances, response to certain drugs, and association with other putative immunopathological diseases of the skin, eye and joints, make it seem probable that in Crohn's disease the intestinal wall is being damaged by an immunological process.

Mode of Tissue Damage

There are four types of immunological reaction (Gell and Coombs, 1968) which, singly or in combination, can cause tissue damage—

Type I, in which IgE affects mast cells to release histamine and other substances which give an anaphylactoid reaction. This acute type of phenomenon is unlikely in Crohn's disease.

Type II, where antibody and antigen react, with the participation of complement, causing lysis of bacteria and other cell damage. Again, this is not likely to be the *main* cause of tissue damage in Crohn's disease.

Type III, in which there is increased permeability of the endothelium, allowing circulating antibodies to enter the walls of blood vessels and react with antigens and so activate complement. Vasculitis produces erythema nodosum in the skin. This type III reaction, when very prolonged, produces follicular, granulomatous lesions, as in farmer's lung. The type III reaction may coexist with type IV.

Type IV is the cell-mediated immunological reaction.

The damage to the intestinal wall in Crohn's disease is probably the result of a type III or type IV reaction, or a combination of both—if indeed an immunopathological process is to blame. Local tissue destruction may release more antigen, and the process become self-perpetuating. Damage might allow extraneous antigen to enter the tissues from the lumen of the intestine. The surgeon's knife may excise the damaged tissue; it cannot hope to eradicate the long immunological memory. Years after an apparently successful resection some minor traumatic lesion to the mucosa or alteration in intestinal flora may reactivate that memory.

Discussion

The hypothesis put forward here that Crohn's disease may be caused by an immunopathological reaction is not incompatible with the observed facts and the hypotheses mentioned earlier in this chapter. Heredity and stress may alter immunological reactivity. Many bacterial components can have an adjuvant action in increasing an immunological reaction. Some component of the dead bacteria could conceivably play a part in the aetiology of Crohn's disease.

Ingested irritants may induce a state of hypersensitivity, possibly after being altered by bacterial action. There might even be several types of reaction to different components within one irritant. With a powerful antigen–antibody reaction in the local segment of ileum it is not surprising that mesenteric adenitis and lymphoedema are among the earliest macroscopic features of Crohn's disease. The fluctuating course of the disease may be the result either of variations in the immune responsiveness of the patient or of periodic alterations in the antigenic challenge such as changes in the degradation of ingested antigens within the bowel and in their rate of absorption.

No satisfactory explanation has ever been advanced for the presence of "skip areas" in a few patients with Crohn's disease. Indeed it is surprising that if the immunological system has been sensitized to recognize some component of intestinal wall as "non-self" that the whole length of the intestine is not involved by the disease. Skip lesions may only appear at places where local resistance or tolerance is reduced. Some normal human alpha-globulins (symbodies) may have immuno-suppressive powers, and be able to protect parts of the intestine (Fink, 1970). It is a feature of some immunological diseases such as erythema nodosum that much of the tissue which is affected appears quite normal, he lesions being confined to a few restricted areas.

References

Adsersen, V. (1931), *Mskr. Dyrlaeg.*, **44**, 465.
Aluwihare, A. P. R. (1970), *Proc. Roy. Soc. Med.*, **64**, 162.
Arapov, D. A., Rolshtchikov, I. M. and Strelnikov, B. E. (1971), *Chir. Gastroent.*, **5**, 272.
Aries, V., Crowther, J. S., Drasar, B. S. and Hill, M. J. (1969), *Gut*, **10**, 575.
Asherson, G. L. (1967), *Brit. med. J.*, **2**, 479.
Aubrey, D. A. (1970), *Arch. Surg. (Chicago)*, **100**, 144.
Bell, H. G. (1934), *Calif. West. Med.*, **41**, 239.
Bendizen, G., Jarnum, S., Soltoft, J., Westergaard, H., Weeke, B. and Yssing, M. (1968), *Scand. J. Gastroent.*, **3**, 481.
Bendixen, G. (1969), *Gut*, **10**, 631.
Bianco, G. (1966), *Ann. Ital. Chir.*, **42**, 1118.
Binder, H., Spiro, H. and Thayer, W. (1966), *Amer. J. Digest. Dis.*, **11**, 572.
Bockus, H. L. and Lee, W. E. (1935), *Ann. Surg.*, **102**, 412.
Bockus, H. L. (1945), *J. Amer. med. Ass.*, **127**, 449.
Brobergerer, O. and Perlmann, P. (1959), *J. Expt. Med.*, **110**, 657.
Cambell, P. G. and Shaw, D. G. (1966), *Brit. med. J.*, **2**, 524.

Cartensen, J. and Poulsen, E. (1971). *Food Additives and Food Contaminants in Regional Enteritis (Crohn's Disease)*. Stockholm: Skandia International Symposia.
Chalfin, D. and Holt, P. R. (1967), *Amer. J. Digest. Dis.*, **12**, 81.
Chess, S., Orlander, G., Puestow, C. B., Benner, W. and Chess, D. (1950), *Surg. Gynec. Obstet.*, **91**, 343.
Christensen, N. (1969), *Amer. J. Surg.*, **118**, 612.
Clark, R. M. (1970), *Canad. med. Ass. J.*, **103**, 24.
Corlin, R. F. and Pops, M. A. (1971), *Gastroenterology*, **60**, 652.
Crockett, R. W. (1952), *Lancet*, **1**, 946.
Debray, C. (1969), *Presse Med.*, **77**, 1307.
Dobbins, W. L. (1966), *Gastroenterology*, **51**, 994.
Drasar, B. S. and Shiner, M. (1969), *Gut*, **10**, 812.
Edwards, H. (1969), *Ann. roy. Coll. Surg. Eng.*, **44**, 121.
Emsbo, P. (1951), *Nord. vet. med.*, **3**, 1.
Feldman, F., Cantor, D., Soll, S. and Bachrach, W. (1967), *Brit. med. J.*, **4**, 711.
Felsen, J. (1936), *Amer. J. Digest. Dis.*, **3**, 86.
Fiedling, J. F. (1970), *Lancet*, **2**, 424.
Fink, S. (1970), *Gastroenterology*, **59**, 334.
Fletcher, J. and Hinton, J. M. (1967), *Lancet*, **2**, 753.
Geffroy, Y., Colin, R. and Charvet, P. (1970), *Arch. Franc. Med. App. Digest*, **59**, 157.
Gell, P. G. H. and Coombs, R. R. A. (1968), *Clinical Aspects of Immunology*. Oxford: Blackwell.
Ghoos, Y. and Vantrappen, G. (1970), *Gastroenterology*, **58**, 951.
Goldberg, D. (1970), *Gut*, **11**, 459.
Golde, D. W. (1968), *Lancet*, **1**, 1144.
Gorbach, S., Nahas, L., Plaut, A., Weinstein, L., Patterson, J. and Levitan, R. (1968), *Gastroenterology*, **54**, 575.
Gorbach, S. and Tabaqchali, S. (1969), *Gut*, **10**, 963.
Hammer, R., Ashurst, P. and Naish, J. (1968), *Gut*, **9**, 17.
Harrison, W. T. (1965), Personal communication.
Jensen, K. B., Goltermann, N., Jarnum, S., Weeke, B. and Westergaard, H. (1970), *Gut*, **11**, 223.
Jones, F. A. and Gummer, P. (1960), *Clinical Gastroenterology*. Oxford: Blackwell.
Jones, J. V., Housley, J., Ashurst, P. M. and Hawkins, C. F. (1969), *Gut*, **10**, 52.
Kalima, T. V. and Collan, Y. (1970), *Scand. J. Gastroent.*, **5**, 497.
Katsaros, D. and Truelove, S. C. (1969), *New Engl. J. Med.*, **281**, 295.
Kennedy, P. C. and Cello, R. M. (1966), *Gastroenterology*, **51**, 926.
Koffler, D., Minkowitz, S., Rothman, W. and Garlock, J. (1962), *Amer. J. Path.*, **41**, 733.
Kyle, J., Bell, T. M., Ponteous, I. B., Blair, D. W. (1963), *Bull. Soc. Int. Clin.* **22**, 575.
Lennard-Jones, J. E. and Morson, B. C. (1969), *D.M.*, **1**, 37.
McBride, J., King, M., Baikie, A., Crean, G. and Sircus, W. (1963), *Brit. med. J.*, **2**, 483.
McMahon, A. W., Patterson, J. F. and Schmitt, P. (1971), *Gastroenterology*, **60**, 696.
Maratka, M. Z. (1961), *Arch. mal. appar. digest.*, **50**, 1263.
Marcus, R. and Watt, J. (1969), *Lancet*, **2**, 489.
Mitchell, D. N., Cannon, P., Dyer, N. H., Hinson, K. F. W. and Willoughby, J. M. T. (1969), *Lancet*, **2**, 571.
Mitchell, D. N. and Rees, R. J. W. (1970), *Lancet*, **2**, 168.
Morganroth, J. and Watson, D. W. (1970), *Amer. J. Dig. Dis.*, **15**, 653.
Morlock, C., Bargen, J. and Pemberton, J. (1939), *Proc. Mayo Clin.*, **14**, 631.
Phear, D. N. (1958), *Lancet*, **2**, 1250.
Pinedo, G. and Watson, D. W. (1971), *Gastroenterology*, **60**, 706.

Prohaska, J. (1966), *Gastroenterology*, **51**, 913.
Reichert, F. L. and Mathes, M. E. (1936), *Ann. Surg.*, **104**, 601.
Reinhart, J. and Succop, R. (1968), *J. Child Psychiat.*, **7**, 258.
Sanders, R. (1964), *Gut*, **5**, 194.
Schmidt, G. T., Lennard-Jones, J., Morson, B. C. and Young, A. C. (1968), *Gut*, **9**, 7.
Schneierson, S. S., Garlock, J. H., Shore, B., Stuart, W. D., Steinglass, M. and Aronson, B. (1962), *Amer. J. Digest. Dis.*, **7**, 839.
Schofield, P. F., Deodhar, S. D. and Turnbull, R. (1969), *Roy. Coll. Surg. Edin.*, **14**, 157.
Sheehan, R. G. (1967), *New Engl. J. Med.*, **277**, 1124.
Shorter, R. G., Cardoza, M. R., ReMine, S. G., Spencer, R. J. and Huizenga, K. A. (1970), *Gastroenterology*, **58**, 692.
Sinaiko, E. S., Nechezes, H. and Greene, V. J. (1946), *Surgery*, **20**, 395.
Slaney, G. (1962), *Ann. Roy. Coll. Surg. Eng.*, **31**, 249.
Smith, F. (1969), *Aust. N.Z. J. Surg.*, **38**, 199.
Solomons, G. F. (1969), *Ann. N.Y. Acad. Sci.*, **164**, 335.
Söltoft, J. (1969), *Scand. J. Gastroent.*, **4**, 353.
Strande, A., Sommers, S. C., Petrak, M. (1954), *Arch. Path.*, **57**, 357.
Struthers, J., Singleton and Kern, F. (1965), *Ann. Intern. Med.*, **63**, 221.
Tabaqchali, S. (1970), *Scand. J. Gastroent.*, Suppl. 6, 139.
Taylor, K., Truelove, S. and Wright, R. (1964), *Gastroenterology*, **46**, 99.
Thayer, W., Brown, M., Sangree, M., Katz, J. and Hersh, T. (1969), *Gastroenterology*, **57**, 311.
Tomasi, T. B., Tan, E. M., Solomon, A. and Prendergast, R. A. (1965), *J. Expt. Med.*, **121**, 101.
Tomenius, J., Larre, E., Lindgren, I., Blumenthal, B. and Lindewall, G. (1963), *Gastroenterologica*, **99**, 368.
Tomenius, J. (1969), in *Modern Gastroenterology*. Eds. O. Gregor and O. Ried, p. 903. Stuttgart and New York: Schattauer Verlag.
Weeke, B. and Jarnum, S. (1971), *Gut*, **12**, 297.
Wells, C. (1952), *Ann. Roy. Coll. Surg. Eng.*, **11**, 105.
Whybrow, P. C., Kane, F. J. and Lipton, M. A. (1968), *Brit. med. J.*, **1**, 708.
Williams, W. J. (1965), *Gut*, **6**, 503.
Willoughby, J. M. T. and Mitchell, D. N. (1971), *Brit. med. J.*, **3**, 155.
Winblad, S., Nilehn, B. and Sternby, N. (1966), *Lancet*, **2**, 1363.

Chapter IV
Pathology

The surgeon is interested in the pathology of Crohn's disease for two main reasons—so that he will recognize the condition when he encounters it and so as to be able to relate the pathologist's report with the clinical state of the patient. Like the physician and the experimental worker in gastroenterology, the abdominal surgeon hopes to learn more about the aetiology and progression of Crohn's disease by detailed light and electron-microscopy studies on resected or biopsy specimens.

There is no room for complacency about the recognition macroscopically of Crohn's disease. Surgeons in Britain did not recognize colonic involvement for 20 years after the disease was first described (Wells, 1952). It was several decades before it was realized that a fistula-in-ano might antedate an overt lesion in the intestine by several years (Morson and Lockhart-Mummery, 1959). In 1972 Crohn's disease in an unusual site is likely to mystify even an experienced abdominal surgeon for a time.

Microscopy, although a most useful method for excluding other causes of granulomatous lesions in the intestine, for example tuberculosis or actinomycosis, has not advanced knowledge about the aetiology of Crohn's disease as much as might have been anticipated. The findings on histological examination do not make it clear whether Crohn's disease is a single entity or a group of conditions resulting from several different agents and pathological processes. The appearances are currently regarded as being compatible with some unusual immunological reaction, but they could be the end-product of some other biological phenomenon.

Probably too much attention has been paid in the past to the end-product. All routine and most research pathology studies tend to concentrate on the worst affected part of the intestine, as it is assumed that the diagnosis will be established most quickly and with the highest degree of certainty by taking sections through the deepest ulcer, the thickest part of the wall, or the largest lymph node. This may or may not be true for diagnosis, but this type of examination is most unlikely to throw much new light on the early stages of the disease when aetiological clues are more likely to be discerned. Very little attention has been directed towards changes at the proximal (or distal) end of a Crohn's lesion or to adjacent normal looking intestine. Few resected specimens have been pinned out and had a systematic study made of bowel and related lymph nodes at all levels. The earliest lesions would appear to be the most hopeful field for investigation. The causes of wars are rarely found in the middle of scarred battlefields.

The forces of destruction and of repair may have been doing battle with one another for some years before the piece of affected intestine is submitted to the pathologist. Medical therapy may possibly have had some effect on the histological appearances. It is not surprising that the pathologist has difficulty in deciding through what stages a lesion has passed. Several workers (Warren and Sommers, 1948; Meadows and Batsakis, 1963) have attempted to define phases through which the diseases may progress, but have not related these phases to the length of history or severity of symptoms at the time of resection. Crohn's disease occurs most frequently in the terminal part of the ileum, one of the most difficult parts of the body to biopsy. Serial biopsy studies of ileal disease are not possible. However, with the rising incidence of colonic disease and the introduction of flexible endoscopes, it should be possible to obtain biopsies at regular intervals from patients with Crohn's disease of colon and rectum. Sequential studies may provide a better understanding of the cellular reaction.

In most specimens the morphological appearances are probably an admixture of a primary and fundamental reaction with a secondary reaction resulting from ulceration and invasion of the wall by intestinal bacteria. Part of a specimen may show late and advanced changes, while another part of the same specimen, or a skip lesion, may reveal much earlier changes. The latter may be found in a recurrence after operation for an advanced lesion. Because of the considerable merging and overlapping, Meadows and Batsakis (1963) felt that the histological appearances should be regarded as a spectrum; a cellular picture which lay within this spectrum would be compatible with the diagnosis of Crohn's disease.

Site of Crohn's Disease

In the Aberdeen series, the small intestine was the part of the alimentary tract primarily affected in most cases; in only 33 out of the 166 patients was the large bowel the principal site of disease. However, in some patients both parts were affected. When there is chronic Crohn's disease in the terminal ileum it is common for the part of the caecum immediately adjacent to be thickened and inflamed; there were 28 cases in this category in Aberdeen. A further 17 patients had more marked caecal involvement; the granulomatous process had extended into the appendix in most of this group. In 3 cases Crohn's disease first appeared in the appendix, only manifesting itself elsewhere in 2 of them after some months or years (Ewen *et al.*, 1971). Altogether 73 patients (44 per cent) had Crohn's lesions in some part of the large bowel (including caecum and rectum). Gross changes were present in the rectum and anal canal of 18 patients, but in half of these there were, or had been earlier, Crohn's lesions at more proximal sites in the intestine (Kyle *et al.*, 1969).

The name "terminal ileitis" is not popular in Britain and is not euphonious, but it is true that most Crohn's lesions are located in the distal part of the ileum. Of the 133 patients with predominantly small bowel involvement in the Aberdeen series, the disease appeared at operation or on X-ray to be in the terminal ileum and to reach the ileo-caecal valve in 114. Eleven patients had Crohn's disease at a more proximal level of the ileum with a length of apparently healthy bowel between the distal macroscopic limit of disease and the caecum. The jejunum was involved in 7 patients but was confined to it in only 2. One example of Crohn's disease of the pyloric antrum and first part of the duodenum was observed.

Discontinuity is one of the more characteristic features of Crohn's disease of the colon, so that the number of multiple lesions there means little. When the colon is not involved, and Crohn's disease is present only in the small intestine, skip lesions are not as common as is sometimes suggested. In the 93 Aberdeen patients with small bowel disease, skip lesions more than 10 cm away from the main lesion were noted in 7 (8 per cent), and in 5 of these the skip lesions were multiple.

The sites of disease in north-east Scotland correspond closely with those noted in the Uppsala region of central Sweden (Krause *et al.*, 1971). In a clinical series totalling 186 patients, there were 77 patients (41·5 per cent) in whom the colon was affected. Among the 109 patients with mainly small bowel disease, the lesion was proximal to the terminal ileum in 10 and in the jejunum in 7 patients in the Swedish series.

Reports which appeared before 1960 contain few cases with Crohn's disease of the colon, so that comparison is more difficult. In the Mayo Clinic series (van Patter *et al.*, 1954), more than half the cases were confined to the terminal ileum and in these the adjacent caecum and ascending colon were also involved in 34 per cent of cases. The middle and upper ileum were the site of disease in 3 per cent and the jejunum in 6·5 per cent, but in some of these patients the disease straddled the somewhat arbitrary boundary line between the two major parts of the small intestine. The Boston workers (Warren and Sommers, 1948) recorded an incidence of jejunal disease of 4 per cent. Ileal disease had spread to the right colon in 15 per cent of their patients. Skip areas were detected in 9 per cent of the Boston patients and in 9·6 per cent of those from the Mayo Clinic.

To summarize, in 1972 the ileum is still by far the commonest site of Crohn's disease. Two patients out of five will have disease in their large bowel, but in only half this number will the large bowel be the main structure attacked by the granulomatous process. Only one patient in 20 will have jejunal disease, and only one patient in 12 will have a skip lesion some distance away in the small intestine.

Macroscopic Appearance

Several colourful terms have been applied to Crohn's disease. Dalziel (1913) described the chronic ileal form of the disease as looking like "an eel in a state of rigor mortis". Apart from the fact that not every surgeon will be well acquainted with dead eels, the macroscopic appearances almost certainly vary with the duration and the degree of activity of the inflammation in the bowel wall.

Small Bowel

With the common type of chronic lesion in the lower ileum the outside diameter of the thickened wall is mostly increased, and may be about 3 cm. The wall itself is often 1 cm thick. However, in some patients the overall diameter does not exceed that of normal ileum, being 1·5–2 cm across. These patients are likely to have more stenotic lesions which are probably of relatively long duration. It is not uncommon to find skip areas higher up the small intestine which appear narrower on the outside than does the adjacent bowel.

The length of ileum showing gross evidence of Crohn's disease varies greatly. In most instances it will lie between 15 cm and 25 cm and demarcation from normal bowel is clear. Some unfortunate patients have long lengths of small intestine involved. Resected specimens have measured up to 150 cm (usually measured after fixation, which causes shrinkage). However, surgeons are aware that on rare occasions virtually the whole small intestine appears more or less unhealthy and no resection is possible; the severity of the granulomatous reaction may vary in different parts.

The other difficult group from the point of view of making a diagnosis at laparotomy are the patients in whom only a narrow, short, strictured area, perhaps 1·5 cm long, is found. There is always the suspicion that such a localized lesion is the end result of a solitary ulcer on the mucosa or of compression from without by a band or the neck of a hernial sac, damaging the wall. This type of short segment is very liable to cause intestinal obstruction; the bowel proximal to it is frequently dilated. Longer, thickened, tortuous segments of bowel with Crohn's disease are often associated with some degree of subacute obstruction, and when the disease has been present for years pseudo-diverticula may be seen proximal to the main mass.

The serosal surface of the ileum has a matt appearance, and may be somewhat wrinkled. With early and active disease the colour is purplish, but later it becomes whiter, although there may always be some injected areas. Foreshortening of the wall produces a concertina-like or contorted effect. Rarely a very few white or grey nodules, 2–3 mm in diameter may be noted on the serosal aspect, which are probably caused by cellular aggregates or, less likely, by blocked lacteals. It is fanciful to refer to this appearance as miliary Crohn's disease; it bears no resemblance to miliary tuberculosis as it was seen within the peritoneal cavity 25 to 30 years ago.

The affected bowel feels sodden and heavy. On palpation the change to normal bowel can be quite noticeable and sharp although sometimes the transition is more gradual. The thickened wall will not indent with the fingers, feeling almost like cartilage in places, particularly in skip lesions, and if flexed acutely will split open. Unfortunately, inspection and palpation are not entirely reliable methods of deciding the upper limit of disease; on transecting the bowel and opening the ends submucous oedema and tiny mucosal ulcers may be detected in parts that were thought to be healthy. These punctate apthoid ulcers overlie lymphocytic aggregates.

Mesentery
Warren and Sommers (1948) stated that the mesentery was uniformly thickened. While it is often true that the mesentery of the lower ileum s so thickened as to constitute a serious embarrassment to the surgeon, in some patients with undoubted Crohn's disease it may be thin and almost transparent, or only show patchy areas of thickening. Oedema and thickening up to 3 cm deep suggests that the mesentery subtends an area of very active inflammation in the bowel wall. This is probably correct but it does not seem to influence the long-term results of resection through this rather dangerous type of mesentery. When the mesentery is thick, fat mostly encroaches onto the ileal wall and in places claw-like processes of fat may almost encircle it.

Lymph Nodes
The dimensions of the lymph nodes are as variable as those of the mesentery that contains them. In a thick mesentery there may be nodes up to 3 cm in diameter, often close together and extending into the root and retroperitoneum. However, there can be pathologically enlarged nodes in a mesentery that otherwise appears normal. In some patients with marked changes in the ileal wall the related lymph nodes look normal. Three adult patients have been seen who presented as suspected appendicitis. At laparotomy only a marked adenopathy of the glands in the ileo-caecal angle was found. Histological examination of the appendices that were removed showed only a few round cells in the wall. Between 1 and 4 years later each of these patients developed typical Crohn's disease of the terminal ileum. Idiopathic mesenteric adenopathy is unusual in an adult and to a surgeon it seems possible that the gland enlargement in these 3 patients bore some relationship to their subsequent Crohn's disease.

Occasionally a calcified lymph gland is detected, but the incidence is probably no higher than in the general population. Calcification does not rule out the possibility of Crohn's disease. While the cause of the early glandular enlargement is unknown, it is likely that in at least a few of the more advanced cases secondary infection may be responsible. It is surprising that more abscesses do not form in these infected nodes; there were only two mesenteric gland abscess in the Aberdeen series.

Adhesions

Long-standing inflammation in the ileum might be expected to give rise to troublesome adhesions. However, in half the cases the affected segment is remarkably mobile, a fact which can cause difficulty with diagnosis but renders resection easier. Warren and Sommers (1948) noted adhesions in 26 per cent of cases. Usually adhesions are between adjacent loops of ileum or to the apex of the sigmoid colon. Internal fistulae may tether a further 15–20 per cent of diseased loops, and in a few patients an ileo-caecal mass is densely adherent to the front of the ilio-psoas sheath.

In Crohn's disease the adhesions are not always simple bands of fibrous tissue. When a sigmoid loop has to be resected along with lower ileum, on histological examination the colon may reveal a typical granulomatous reaction even though no fistula has been present.

Colon and Rectum

In general Crohn's disease of the large bowel presents a similar external appearance to that described in the ileum, but it may be partially hidden by great omentum and appendices epiploicae. The fixed positions of the ascending colon, splenic flexure and descending colon make these parts more difficult to inspect thoroughly, and their related lymph nodes are not so accessible as those in the mesentery.

Long lengths, 30–50 cm, of colon may be uninterruptedly thickened and diseased. Subserosal vascular injection is frequently prominent. More mobile parts, such as the transverse colon, feel heavy, indurated and inelastic. The sensation is quite different to the flaccid insipid feeling that typical idiopathic ulcerative proctocolitis imparts to palpating fingers. Discontinuity and asymmetry are characteristic features of Crohn's disease of the colon. On opening the abdomen it may be obvious at once that the sigmoid loop is reddened, thickened and oedematous, that its serosa has lost its sheen. Then after palpating along normal descending colon thick longitudinal patches are discovered in the transverse colon; they feel not unlike an extra and grossly thickened taenia on the colon. Finally a lesion may be found in the ileo-caecal valve. There was one example of Crohn's disease initially localized to the valve in the Aberdeen series.

When the rectum is the site of Crohn's disease the mucosa at first looks red and friable when viewed through a sigmoidoscope. Although the superficial appearance might be regarded as that of non-specific proctitis, rectal biopsy often reveals a granulomatous reaction (Dyer *et al.*, 1970). The inflammation can progress rapidly—within a few weeks or months the lumen may be narrowed and distorted. Tumour-like masses may be palpable and a rectal stricture is not uncommon. A very high proportion of patients with Crohn's disease in the distal colon and rectum have perianal lesions—recurrent abscesses, fistulae-in-ano, indolent ulcers or painless fissures on the anal verge. Histo-logical examination of tissue excised from the perianal region will in many instances show granulomas and giant cells, but inevitably there is considerable super-added infection.

Mucosal Appearance

When a resected specimen of terminal ileum is opened, the mucosal appearance may be rather disappointing to anyone expecting wide-spread ulceration. Instead, one part of the surface may look normal while another part is composed of small mounds of somewhat oedematous mucosa, commonly 4–6 mm across. Packed together they do bear some resemblance to cobblestones, albeit of a rather coarse type. It is not a very common appearance. Between the mounds there are intersecting, fine linear ulcers, or deep fissures. The depths of these clefts cannot be clearly seen in many parts of any one specimen, but here and there ulcers are present. Such ulcers are said to be more common on the mesenteric side of the ileum. However, most specimens are opened along their anti-mesenteric border and ulcers on this side might be bisected and be less obvious when the rather rigid specimen is opened out.

Among the resected specimens in Aberdeen, ulceration was more extensive when Crohn's disease was present in the more proximal part of the ileum or in the jejunum. Here, in some patients, there were large ulcerated areas. The floor of these denuded areas was composed of a cream-coloured, tenacious slough, reminiscent of the now largely for-gotten diphtheritic membrane. Not surprisingly these were the patients who manifested a protein-losing enteropathy.

Around the larger lumen of the colon, the islets or mounds of mucosa are also larger. Where ulcers are obvious there is more tendency for them to be longitudinal, often extending over distances of several centimetres. At intervals these long, straight ulcers may be connected by cross-clefts, giving a railway track appearance. The most unusual ulcers in the Aberdeen series were seen in the rectum. Here there were discrete, flat, ovoid ulcers up to 2 cm long, with a purple or red edge and base, and separated from each other by areas of mucosa that looked normal or only showed a fine cobblestone pattern.

Many patients with colonic Crohn's disease are over the age of 50 years, and so are liable to have diverticula present in the distal part of the colon. However, if Crohn's disease is present it is almost impossible to demonstrate the orifice of any diverticulum on the mucosal surface. The full thickness of the colon wall and any diverticula are all involved in the granulomatous process. Inflammation may spread into the pericolic tissues (Lockhart-Mummery and Morson, 1964).

Histology of Chronic Crohn's Disease

For more than 20 years in Britain the study carried out by Hadfield in 1939 was regarded as the definitive work on the pathology of Crohn's disease. It was the yardstick used by most pathologists to make the diagnosis. Some used it too rigorously, and from Hadfield's observations developed and adopted strict criteria that he himself had never laid down. During those years some resected specimens were reported as non-specific granuloma, chronic inflammation, atypical or non-caseating tuberculosis simply because they did not show every one of the features that Hadfield mentioned in his paper. It was only after the unfortunate patients had undergone numerous operations, developed multiple fistulae, and the whole sad clinical saga was reviewed in retrospect, that the correct diagnosis was made. It was then a clinical diagnosis overriding the original pathology report which had by implication, if not in as many words, excluded Crohn's disease.

Because of the misunderstanding that it sometimes caused and the way that it was interpreted, it is worthwhile both reviewing what Hadfield actually wrote and seeing how closely his findings agree with 1972 views on the microscopic appearances of Crohn's disease.

In 1939 abdominal tuberculosis was still common and colonic involvement by Crohn's disease was not generally recognized. Hadfield studied only 20 cases, a small number by 1972 standards, but relatively large for 1939. All 20 patients had ileal disease; in 17 (85 per cent) the terminal ileum and adjacent caecum were involved, while in 3 the granulomatous process was confined to the lower ileum. The average length of ileum affected was 19 cm, with a range of 4 cm to 60 cm. Seven of the patients had either internal or external fistulae.

The features which Hadfield described in some detail were—

1. Thickening of the ileal wall, visible to the naked eye;
2. Mucosal ulceration, variable in extent and depth;
3. Submucosal lesion, which had 4 components;
4. Regional lymphadenopathy, again somewhat variable.

1. *Thickening of the Wall*—Hadfield described this as a constant and striking feature of the diseased ileum which sharply demarcated it from proximal healthy intestine. Most of the thickening was attributed to changes in the submucous layer. Hypertrophy of muscle was variable, inconstant and regarded as a late feature of the condition. Chronic inflammatory cell infiltration through all layers of the bowel wall was not specifically mentioned.

All subsequent workers are agreed that there is marked thickening of the wall (Warren and Sommers, 1948; Rappaport *et al.*, 1951; van Patter *et al.*, 1954; Morson, 1968). Most agree that it is the swelling in the submucosa that accounts for the major part of the thickening, and that this swelling occurs before there is any breach in the intestinal mucosa (Lewin and Swales, 1966). Oedema in the lamina propria in the submucosa and lymphatic dilatation are often marked (Fig. 1). It is doubtful just how much changes in the muscle layers contribute to the altered dimensions of the wall. Fragmentation in the muscularis mucosae has been described (Meadows and Batsakis, 1963). What looks like

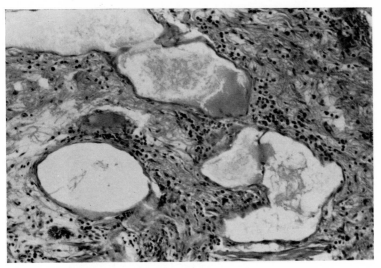

Fig. 1. Histology of Crohn's disease. The lymphoedema and dilatation of lymphatics seen here are among the earliest changes. × 250.

thickening in the muscularis propria may be the result of shortening of the bowel, bunching up the muscle. Warren and Sommers (1948) did regard it as being truly hypertrophied. Lockhart-Mummery and Morson (1964) noted that when diverticula were present in the colon, the muscle layers had an irregular corrugated appearance. Attempts at healing after years of chronic inflammation are bound to alter the configuration of the muscle.

The most important addition to Hadfield's description is the emphasis now placed on the transmural nature of the inflammation (Morson, 1968). Very few other diseases can bring about such changes in all layers of the intestinal wall. Cellular infiltration may be most obvious in the loose tissues of the submucosa but in an established case it can be detected right through to the serosa and even into the mesentery or pericolic tissues. The infiltrate contributes materially to the rigidity and overall thickness.

2. *Ulceration*—While ulceration was noted at some point on the mucosal surface of all specimens, Hadfield pointed out that there could be large areas with intact mucosa, although with considerable swelling in the submucosa. Sometimes ulceration was superficial; in other cases it was deep and gave rise to small abscesses in the wall. Fissures were

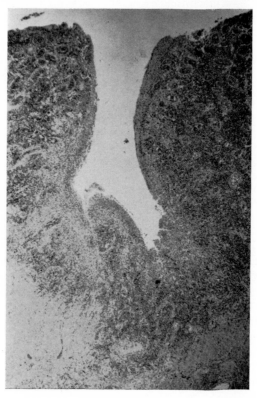

FIG. 2. Fissure formation. The fissure starts on the ulcerated surface of the ileum and is extending deeply into the wall, which is heavily infiltrated with inflammatory cells. × 125.

also noted which Hadfield referred to as perforations, but from his description it is clear that he was observing points of deep penetration into and occasionally through all layers of the wall—in this sense there was transmural inflammation in his specimens.

In the absence of granulomas, these deep fissures (Fig. 2) are the next best criterion for establishing a diagnosis of Crohn's disease (Lockhart-Mummery and Morson, 1964). Crypt abscesses and small intramural abscesses do occur. If enough sections are cut these abscesses will be found to communicate through a fissure or crevice with the lumen.

Recent workers have added little to our knowledge of the ulcers. It has been suggested that they occur at the tops or bottom of folds because of the deformation forces acting there (Amman and Bockus, 1961). The relative degree of immobility provided by the mesentery has been blamed for ulcers being (allegedly) more common on that side of the lumen. As the antimesenteric side may have a slightly poorer blood supply, ulcers might have been expected to appear there. On the other hand there may be less tendency for oedema to collect on the anti-mesenteric side; most workers believe that it is the subjacent oedema that eventually leads to ulceration of the mucosa.

3. *Components in the Submucosal Lesion of Crohn's Disease*—In Hadfield's description the swelling in the submucosa was attributed to obstructive lymphoedema, chronic inflammatory cell infiltrate, hyperplasia of the lymphoid tissue and a granulomatous reaction of what he considered to be endothelial cells along with Langhans-type giant cells. It is clear that Hadfield believed that hyperplasia of pale-staining reticulum cells first occurred in the germinal centres of the lymphoid tissue. In a variable number of these germinal centres, pro-liferating endothelial cells replaced the centre, and formed a cell mass that grew irregularly until all the surrounding lymphocytes had dis-appeared. At this stage two or three Langhans giant cells would be present. Later the endothelial cells retrogressed, becoming attenuated, with more reticulin present, but without marked fibrous tissue for-mation. Sommers and Warren (1948) thought that the endothelial cells came from the lining of the lymphatics.

Today the endothelial cells are called epithelioid; fusion of some of these cells may form the Langhans giant cells, which tend to be pear-shaped with peripherally situated nuclei. Foreign-body giant cells are more circular, with nuclei nearer the centre. The aggregation of epithe-lioid cells and giant cells is usually referred to as a sarcoid reaction (Fig. 3), less often as a tuberculoid reaction. Hadfield himself stated that the appearances were more like those of sarcoid then tuberculosis, and advised prolonged follow-up of patients to exclude sarcoidosis. This has now been done and patients initially diagnosed as Crohn's disease have not developed sarcoidosis elsewhere in the body at a later date. The granulomas are larger, more numerous and lack the surrounding zone of lymphocytes in sarcoidosis.

The sarcoid reaction of Crohn's disease considered by itself, can be virtually indistinguishable from that of tuberculosis (Morson, 1968), but is much less florid in the former disease. In tuberculosis the sub-mucosa is noticeably narrow, not oedematous. Ziehl-Neelsen staining to show up any acid- and alcohol-fast mycobacterium and attempts to

culture the organism by the microbiologist are sometimes necessary
before tuberculosis can be confidently excluded. The granulomas are
rather larger in tuberculosis and more likely to become hyalinized than
they are in Crohn's disease. A sarcoid reaction is also seen in chronic
beryllium disease.

While there are many lymphoid follicles scattered through all layers
of the intestinal wall in Crohn's disease, it is by no means certain that
the sarcoid reaction always starts in a germinal centre, enlarges and then
regresses. There is often lymphoid hyperplasia, and a sarcoid reaction

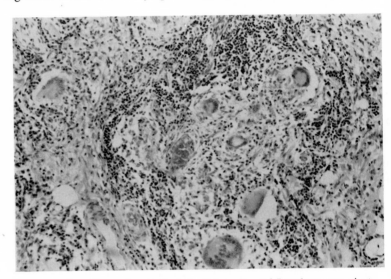

FIG. 3. Sarcoid reaction in Crohn's disease. Several Langhans-type giant
cells are seen among the epithelioid cells, which here are loosely arranged.
A few lymphocytes surround the central granuloma. × 200.

may first be detected in Peyer's patches or other masses of lymphoid
tissue (Rappaport *et al.*, 1951). In a few patients the hyperplasia may be
so great that it simulates a malignant lymphoma. Differentiation can
be difficult (Azzopardi and Menzies, 1959), although in the latter
neoplastic lesion there should be less admixture of cells. However, the
sarcoid reaction in Crohn's disease is found in the muscle layers and
subserosa from which lymphoid tissue is usually absent. The epithelioid
cells may develop from histiocytes or other stem cells. The zone of
lymphocytes that often surrounds the epithelioid cell aggregate may be
a secondary phenomenon.

The relationship of the lymphadenoid and sarcoid foci to blood
vessels is unclear. Morson (1968) considers that they lie near to blood
vessels or to lymphatics in the vicinity of these vessels; Williams (1964)

denies that there is any particular relationship. The compactness of individual sarcoid granulomas and their number vary greatly. In a minority of patients the granulomatous reaction is diffuse; in about 50 per cent it is more focal in type, but in 25–45 per cent no sarcoid reaction can be detected. It is on this last point that Hadfield has most frequently been misinterpreted, although he clearly stated that in 5 cases out of 20 (25 per cent) "all trace of a specific lesion had disappeared". When the sarcoid reaction is absent, the transmural nature of the chronic inflammation and the presence of fissures are the most helpful features in arriving at a correct diagnosis (Morson, 1968). Particularly in the earlier stages of the disease there may be considerable hyperaemia and dilatation of lymphatics. Eosinophils may be seen in the submucosa but in the later stages most of the cells are lymphocytes and plasma cells. In the lamina propria plasma cells are numerous and may appear swollen (Rippey and Sommers, 1968). A few macrophages are present and with special stains PAS positive hyaline material may be demonstrated in them; it could come from an antibody–antigen reaction (Amman and Bockus, 1961). Neutrophil polymorphs are relatively scarce except in the immediate vicinity of ulceration which has entered the submucosa.

A fissure may start close to the edge of an ulcer and extend down to or pass close by a lymphoid follicle (Lockhart-Mummery and Morson, 1964). It is lined by granulation tissue, with polymorphonuclear leucocytes near the surface, and lymphocytes and plasma cells lying deeper. An occasional fissure may extend through the muscle layers and form either a localized abscess or a fistula to another viscus or to the skin.

From the Aberdeen series, 20 resected ileal specimens and 5 colonic specimens were taken at random and the principal histological features noted. There were usually 6 or 8 routine slides available for each specimen; no special sections were cut. The results are given in Table 1. In every patient studied there was transmural inflammation, ulceration of the mucosa at some point and noticeable oedema of the submucosa.

Table 1

Histopathological findings in 25 patients with Crohn's disease

Histological feature	Ileum (20 patients)	Colon (5 patients)	Total
Transmural inflammation	20	5	25 (100%)
Submucosal oedema	20	5	25 (100%)
Ulceration	20	5	25 (100%)
Fissure formation	8	4	12 (48%)
Sarcoid reaction	9	5	14 (56%)
Mucous metaplasia	9	—	9 (45%)
Endarteritis	9	1	10 (40%)

A definite sarcoid reaction was present in 56 per cent of the cases, while 48 per cent showed fissuring. There is little doubt that if many more sections had been cut for each specimen a rather higher percentage of granulomas would have been obtained. As it is, with a routine diagnostic service technique, the incidence of fissure formation is higher than the 25 per cent generally recorded (Williams, 1964; Morson, 1968).

Lymph Nodes—Mesenteric Lymphadenopathy is common. Only a minority of nodes show granulomatous foci, and it is not necessarily the largest nodes that do so (Hadfield, 1939). The epithelioid and giant cell systems enlarge up to about 0·75 mm in diameter. It is possible that this increase in size of some nodes is contemporaneous with hyperplasia of lymphoid tissue in the bowel wall and may even antedate it. Most surgeons submit few enlarged nodes for histopathological examination. This practice is wrong and in part accounts for sarcoid reaction being found in only 20–25 per cent of specimens (Williams, 1964; Lockhart-Mummery and Morson, 1964). The remainder are reported as showing reactive hyperplasia. Some of the normal looking nodes might have contained typical granulomas. Hadfield examined two nodes with a sarcoid reaction when only non-specific changes were detected in the related intestine. One similar example was found in Aberdeen. Morson, who uses the multiple section technique, for the intestine, doubts if this ever happens.

The absence of caseation in lymph nodes is helpful in excluding tuberculosis.

Other Changes

Close to and over the area affected by Crohn's disease the intestinal villi are rather stunted and broader (Amman and Bockus, 1961; Meadows and Batsakis, 1963); the mucosa is thicker but with less tall columnar cells (Madanagopolan *et al.*, 1965). In some patients there may be patches of partial villous atrophy well proximal to the main lesion (Shiner and Drury, 1962). These patches are very irregular in their distribution and a great many suction jejunal biopsies may have to be taken before one is found. The atrophy is never as severe as the sub-total type characteristic of idiopathic steatorrhoea. Dehydrogenase deficiencies have been reported in some intestinal cells (Binder, 1968); the significance, if any, of this variation is not known at present.

Mucous metaplasia of the intestinal glands (Fig. 4) is observed in about half of the patients with chronic ileal disease (Antonius *et al.*, 1960; Ming *et al.*, 1963) and is most noticeable close to ulcerated areas. Depending on the depth to which the clear-looking irregular glands penetrate, the metaplasia may be referred to as pyloric-gland change (common) or Brunner gland changes (deeper and rarer). In most diseases of the small intestine the Paneth cells are decreased in number; in Crohn's disease they are increased (Lewin, 1969).

Hyalinization rarely occurs in the centre of a granuloma. Caseation is never seen, but in 2–3 per cent of cases some epithelioid cells appear to have undergone necrosis.

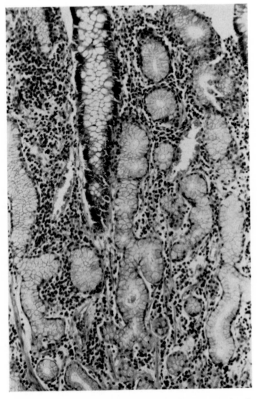

FIG. 4. Mucous metaplasia in the glands of the ileum proximal to an area ulcerated by Crohn's disease. × 125.

Schaumann bodies are a very common finding in sarcoidosis, being present in about 90 per cent of cases; they are said to occur in 60 per cent of patients with chronic beryllium disease (Williams, 1964). However, in Crohn's disease they are uncommon, being noted in no more than 5–10 per cent of cases. Mostly the birefringent crystals or shell-like conchoidal bodies are inside the giant cells. As many patients with Crohn's disease will have had multiple operations in the past, it is important to differentiate the appearance from that of talc or other foreign-body granuloma (Lichtman *et al.*, 1946).

More than one-third of the Aberdeen patients showed some degree of endarteritis in the smaller vessels in the bowel wall (Fig. 5). The change is secondary and non-specific. In most patients it is of little importance, but if pronounced, arterial changes could produce small infarcts, with perforation of the bowel wall (Harjola *et al.*, 1965). Thrombosis in small arteries and veins is surprisingly rare in Crohn's disease, considering the chronicity of the adjacent inflammation. Vascular changes are striking in the skin of patients unlucky enough to develop pyoderma gangrenosum (Bishopric and Bracken, 1964). There is fibrinoid necrosis in the media and fragmentation of the internal elastic lamina, with considerable inflammatory cell infiltrate of the walls of the arterioles.

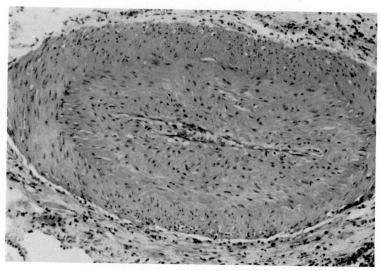

FIG. 5. Endarteritis in an intramural arteriole, from a patient with chronic Crohn's disease of the small intestine. × 250.

The so-called neuromatous appearance is also a secondary and inconstant phenomenon. The apparent increase in nerve elements may result from shortening of the damaged bowel, bringing more ganglion cells and myenteric plexus fibres into a unit area. Oedematous swelling may render them more prominent but the possibility of hyperplasia of neurilemmal cells cannot be completely excluded. Similar appearances are occasionally noted with other forms of chronic ulceration and inflammation, for example, gastric ulcer.

Malignant Tumours Complicating Crohn's Disease of Small Intestine
Adenocarcinoma has been reported with increasing frequency in ileum and jejunum that are the site of Crohn's disease (Shiel *et al.*, 1968;

Wyatt, 1969; Tyers *et al.*, 1969). Sarcoma apparently is rare (Buchanan *et al.*, 1959) although normally it is as common as adenocarcinoma in the small intestine. Among the Aberdeen patients there were two with carcinoid tumours; one was reported as benign, the other as malignant, although none of the other clinical signs and symptoms of a carcinoid syndrome developed.

Crohn's Disease of the Colon

Lockhart-Mummery and Morson (1964) have pointed out that in its pathology Crohn's disease in the large bowel does not differ from that in the ileum, apart from slight variations that the differences in their anatomy and function may impose. Speed of change may be greater in the colon and new lesions are more likely to appear distally rather than proximally (Brahme and Wenckert, 1970). Schaumann bodies are slightly more common in the giant-cells in colon wall and in patients who have fistulae to the skin, for example in the perianal region. An occasional foreign-body giant cell may be seen close to where the mucosa has been breached, or in the lining of a fistula-in-ano.

Histopathological examination is very valuable in differentiating Crohn's disease from ulcerative colitis, diverticulitis, ischaemic disease of the colon and from lymphogranuloma venereum affecting the rectum. Idiopathic ulcerative proctocolitis is essentially a mucosal disease, whereas in Crohn's disease all layers of the colon wall are involved. The lymph nodes in ulcerative colitis are usually small and shotty (Brooke, 1962); they are more likely to be enlarged and to be centrally located in Crohn's disease. The main histological differences between the two diseases are shown in Table 2, which is based on the studies at St

Table 2

Microscopic differences between ulcerative colitis and colonic Crohn's disease

Histological feature	Ulcerative proctocolitis	Crohn's disease of colon
Inflammation	Mucosal	Transmural
Vascularity	Marked	Uncommon
Sarcoid granulomas	Absent	Present
Fissures	Absent	Common
Lymphoid hyperplasia	Mucosal	All coats
Crypt abscess	Common	Rare
Mucus secretion	Greatly decreased	Nearly normal

Mark's Hospital, London (Lennard-Jones *et al.*, 1968). In Crohn's disease the goblet cell population is maintained. The mucin content of the mucosa remains normal, while in ulcerative proctocolitis it is markedly reduced (Hellstrom and Fisher, 1967; Filipe and Dawson,

1970). Using these criteria it is usually possible to separate ulcerative disease of the colon into the two distinct clinico-pathological entities. However, many writers appreciate that in up to 10 per cent of cases clear-cut differentiation is not possible (Hawke and Turnbull, 1966; Lewin and Swales, 1967; Kent *et al.*, 1970).

Toxic dilatation of the colon is a serious complication of ulcerative colitis. The thickened wall of Crohn's disease of the colon might have been expected to prevent such dilatation; nevertheless it does occur, although rarely (Morson, 1966; Javett and Brooke, 1970). Neoplastic change in the colonic mucosa is a well recognized hazard of long-standing ulcerative colitis. The follow-up period in patients with Crohn's disease of the colon is still too short to be able to assess the incidence of colonic cancer or the factors that may influence its onset. Examples are being reported with increasing frequency (Parrish *et al.*, 1968; Jones, 1969; Perret *et al.*, 1968).

The inflammation in diverticulitis is around the bowel wall rather than in it; it is a pericolitis (Schmidt *et al.*, 1968). Diverticula are often present in the descending and sigmoid colon which show involvement by Crohn's disease. It may not be possible to tell the nature of a short strictured area or tumour mass at laparotomy. When Crohn's disease is present, most patients will have rectal involvement which can be seen on sigmoidoscopy or on examining a rectal biopsy specimen; perianal fistulae are very common in these patients.

The splenic flexure has the poorest blood supply of any part of the large or small intestine. There is no reason to doubt that sometimes one of the lengthy, tenuous vessels supplying the flexure may become occluded. Local ischaemia could also be caused by disease of small intramural vessels. The ischaemic portion of wall is said to be infiltrated by granulation tissue, which may contain deposits of haemosiderin; eventually a short stricture forms. If this theory of vascular brinkmanship is correct, it is surprising that no series of gangrenous splenic flexures has been reported that might match the cases being diagnosed as ischaemic colitis.

The distortion that lymphogranuloma venereum sometimes produces in the rectum resembles that of Crohn's disease. Granulomas are found in both conditions. In lymphogranuloma there is frequently necrosis in the centre of the granuloma, which may contain polymorphonuclear leucocytes (Rodaniche *et al.*, 1943). Those acquainted with both diseases have little difficulty in distinguishing them from each other.

The Ultrastructure of the Colon in Crohn's Disease

The best electronmicroscopy study in Crohn's disease is that of Aluwihare (1971). He obtained operation or biopsy specimens from colon and rectum, fixing them at once in 1 per cent osmium tetroxide.

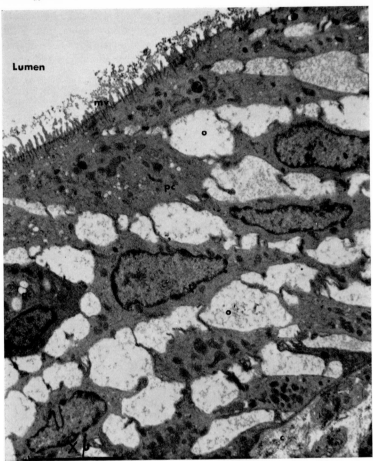

Fig. 6. Electron micrograph of epithelium of the colon in Crohn's disease. The underlying lamina propria is oedematous and infiltrated with lymphocytes and plasma cells. There is marked intercellular oedema (*o*) between the principal cells (*pc*), but the individual cells look normal. (*gc*) = goblet cell; (*mv*) microvilli; (*n*) = nucleus; (*c*) = subepithelial collagen, which is not affected. ×4,200.

The epithelial cells looked remarkably normal, as did their micro-villi. There was some oedema between the cells (Fig. 6) but the under-lying basement membrane and collagen were intact. Numerous plasma cells and lymphocytes were seen in the broadened lamina propria. In ulcerative colitis the epithelial cells, while initially intact, may be smaller with stunted microvilli; there may be a deficiency of collagen and round cell infiltration is less noticeable (Donnallan, 1966). In

Crohn's disease of the colon, Aluwihare found that about 14 per cent of the lymphocyte series had an unduly prominent nucleolus, giving them a cartwheel appearance. They may be undergoing or have been arrested during transformation into plasma cells. Most of the nerve and muscle cells and the blood vessels looked normal.

A special study was made of the epithelioid cells in the granulomas (Fig. 7). They had large nuclei containing finely dispersed chromatin and a clear-cut nucleolus. The close apposition or superimposition of

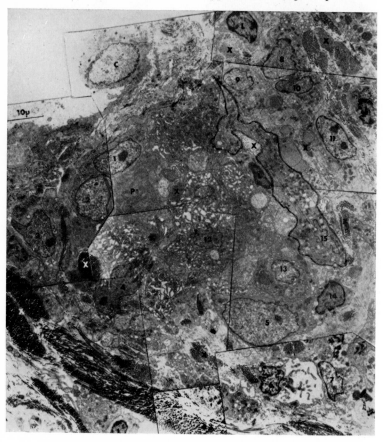

Fig. 7. Montage of electron micrographs of a small epithelioid cell granuloma in the submucosa of the colon. The cells 1–15 were shown to correspond to epithelioid cells in a light micrograph of the adjacent serial section (Aluwihare, 1971). 1–15 = epithelioid cells; L = lymphocytes; P = plasma cell; X = collagen; C = nucleus of endothelial cell of a capillary. The cytoplasm of cell 15 is outlined. Note the close relationship of the epithelioid cells, which have granular chromatin and a prominent nucleolus in their nuclei, to each other and to lymphocytes. ×1,500.

cells can give the appearance of multiple nuclei. The margins between the epithelioid cells were undulating and interdigitating (Fig. 8); there was no true basement membrane present. Towards the periphery of a granuloma, Aluwihare noted that the endoplasmic reticulum of the epithelioid cells was of coarser texture. Nearer the centre, they contained

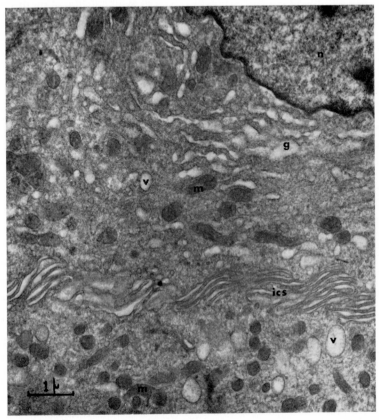

FIG. 8. Adjacent areas of two epithelioid cells. (*n*) = nucleus; (*g*) = golgi zone; (*m*) = mitochondria; (*v*) = vesicles, most of which stain lightly; the endoplasmic reticulum of these cells cannot be seen here. Debris is seen only occasionally. Note the complex filiform interdigitating cell margins (*ics*). × 18,000.

vacuoles. It appeared that these epithelioid cells were metabolically active, possibly forming and storing some protein substance. Few cells contained any debris—phagocytosis did not seem to be their main function.

No specific aetiological agent was detected. Because the epithelial cells were intact, Aluwihare does not consider Crohn's disease of the colon to be primarily an epithelial disease. He regards the changes noted in the lymphocytes, plasma cells and epithelioid cells as being compatible with some immunological reaction.

"Acute Crohn's Disease"

There are probably many different causes of acute inflammation of the terminal ileum, and in only a very few cases is any form of Crohn's disease responsible. In a small number of patients Crohn's disease does present acutely and then progresses into the chronic form already considered. A self-limiting acute form of Crohn's disease is a very doubtful entity.

With the acute onset or self-limiting forms the last 10–15 cm of the ileum are red, swollen and oedematous and there may be free fluid in the peritoneal cavity. Resection is not usually performed unless perforation has taken place. The entire wall is infiltrated with acute inflammatory cells, and there may be some plasma cells and eosinophils; marked hyperaemia is evident (Crohn, 1965; Schofield, 1965). The sarcoid reaction of chronic Crohn's disease is not seen. One of the patients described by Crohn (1965) required a further operation after 9 days and in this short interval typical epithelioid cell granulomas and giant cells had appeared.

In 1966 Fieber and Schaefer presented 4 cases of lymphoid hyperplasia of the terminal ileum. Clinically some of the cases behaved like "acute Crohn's disease". They collected 8 more verified examples from the literature and while the aetiology was unknown, they discussed the possibility of lymphoid hyperplasia being a clinical entity.

Crohn's Disease in Unusual Sites

Meckel's diverticulum is occasionally the site of Crohn's disease, either alone or along with the ileum (Ekman, 1958; Aubrey, 1970). In some of the patients reported the Crohn's disease has been of acute type and there has been perforation of the diverticulum. In Aberdeen only one patient out of 166 had Crohn's disease of the duodenum, but in Birmingham there were 16 examples of duodenal disease in a series of 300 patients (Fielding, 1970). When the lesion is close to the pylorus it may simulate a duodenal ulcer both clinically and at laparotomy. The wall is thick, scarred, looks white and some petechiae may be seen on the serosal surface (Jones *et al.*, 1966; Van der Holden *et al.*, 1969). In most cases Crohn's disease is also present in some other part of the intestinal tract (Edwards *et al.*, 1965).

Gastric involvement is rare. Johnston and his colleagues (1966) have reviewed the literature. The antrum is the part most likely to be affected; in a few cases the whole stomach is involved and externally it closely resembles a leather-bottle stomach (linitis plastica). The pathological features otherwise are the same as those of Crohn's disease in the ileum, with alternating ulceration and hyperplastic mucosa on the inside and a sarcoid-like cellular reaction in the wall. Some typical granulomas have been found within the liver of patients with intestinal disease (Warren and Sommers, 1948) and even the gall-bladder may be involved.

Controversy centres round the condition referred to as regional oesophagitis (Madden *et al.*, 1969). Unlike the stomach and intestine, the oesophagus has a squamous lining. Pope (1970) doubts if the strictures described in the lower oesophagus are in any way connected with Crohn's disease. However, one of the patients reported by Dyer *et al.* (1969) developed Crohn's disease of the ileum shortly afterwards; the dysphagia of which Gelfand and Krone's patient (1969) complained responded to corticosteroids, while Kleineman *et al.* (1970) were able to demonstrate granulomas in an oesophageal biopsy specimen. Several of these patients had had troublesome apthous ulceration of the mouth, a common complication of Crohn's disease. Furthermore it is now recognized that Crohn's lesions can appear in the mouth (Dudeney, 1969) and "metastatic ulceration" of skin may be found in the groins, beneath the breasts and between folds of skin on the abdominal wall (Mountain, 1970). In these latter patients there is well established intestinal disease. Like perinal fistulae, oesophageal strictures may be the harbinger of Crohn's disease that will appear in the bowel at a later date.

References

Aluwihare, A. P. R. (1971), *Proc. Roy. Soc. Med.*, **64**, 162..
Amman, R. W. and Bockus, H. L. (1961), *Arch. Int. Med.*, **107**, 504.
Antonious, J. I., Gump, F. E., Lattes, R. and Lepore, M. (1960), *Gastroenterology*, **38**, 889.
Aubrey, D. A. (1970), *Arch. Surg. (Chicago)*, **100**, 144.
Azzopardi, J. G. and Menzies, T. (1960), *Brit. J. Surg.*, **47**, 358.
Binder, V. (1968), *Scand. J. Gastroent.*, **3**, 611.
Bishopric, G. A. and Bracken, J. S. (1964), *Southern med. J.*, **57**, 675.
Brahme, F. and Wenckert, A. (1970), *Gut*, **11**, 578.
Brooke, B. N. (1962), *Dis. Colon Rectum*, **5**, 138.
Buchanan, D. P., Huebner, G. D., Woolvin, S. C., North, R. L. and Novack, T. D. (1959), *Amer. J. Surg.*, **97**, 336.
Crohn, B. B. (1965), *Amer. J. Digest. Dis.*, **10**, 565.
Dalziel, T. K. (1913), *Brit. med. J.*, **2**, 1068.
Donnellan, W. L. (1966), *Gastroenterology*, **50**, 519.
Dudeney, T. P. (1969), *Proc. Roy. Soc. Med.*, **62**, 1237.
Dyer, N. H., Cook, P. L. and Harper, R. A. K. (1969), *Gut*, **10**, 549.
Dyer, N. H., Stansfeld, A. G. and Dawson, A. M. (1970), *Scand. J. Gastroent.*, **5**, 491.
Edwards, A. M., Michalyshyn, B., Sherbaniuk, R. W. and Costopoulos, L. B. (1965), *Canad. med. Ass. J.*, **93**, 1283.
Ekman, C. N. (1958), *Gastroenterology*, **34**, 130.
Ewen, S. W. B., Anderson, J., Galloway, J. M. D., Miller, J. D. B. and Kyle, J. (1971), *Gastroenterology*, **60**, 853.

Fieber, S. S. and Schaefer, H. J. (1966), *Gastroenterology*, **50**, 83.
Fielding, J. F. (1970), *An Enquiry into Certain Aspects of Regional Enteritis*, M.D. Thesis. National University of Ireland.
Filipe, M. I. and Dawson, I. (1970), *Gut*, **11**, 229.
Gelfand, M. D. and Krone, C. L. (1968), *Gastroenterology*, **55**, 510.
Hadfield, G. (1939), *Lancet*, **2**, 773.
Harjola, P. T., Appelqvist, R. and Lilios, H. G. (1965), *Acta Chir. Scand.*, **130**, 143.
Hawke, W. A. and Turnbull, R. B. (1966), *Gastroenterology*, **51**, 802.
Hellstrom, H. R. and Fisher, E. R. (1967), *Amer. J. Clin. Path.*, **48**, 259.
Javett, S. L. and Brooke, B. N. (1970), *Lancet*, **2**, 126.
Johnson, O. A., Hoskins, D. W., Todd, J. and Thorbjarnarson, B. (1966), *Gastroenterology*, **50**, 571.
Jones, G. W., Dooley, M. R. and Schoenfield, L. J. (1966), *Gastroenterology*, **51**, 1018.
Jones, J. H. (1969), *Gut*, **10**, 651.
Kent, T. H., Ammon, R. K. and Den Besten, L. (1970), *Arch. Path.*, **89**, 20.
Kleinman, M. S., Resnicoff, S. and Wiesner, P. J. (1970), *Gastroenterology*, **58**, 1068.
Krause, U., Bergman, L. and Norlen, B. J. (1971), *Scand. J. Gastroent*, **6**, 97.
Kyle, J., Cole, T. P. and Ewen, S. W. R. (1969), *Prensa med. Argent.*, **56**, 470.
Lennard-Jones, J. E., Lockhart-Mummery, H. E. and Morson, B. C. (1968), *Gastroenterology*, **54**, 1162.
Lewin, K. and Swales, J. D. (1966), *Gastroenterology*, **50**, 211.
Lewin, K. (1969), *Gut*, **10**, 804.
Lichtman, A. L., McDonald, J. R., Dixon, C. F. and Mann, F. C. (1946), *Surg. Gynec. Obstet.*, **83**, 531.
Lockhart-Mummery, H. E. and Morson, B. C. (1964), *Gut*, **5**, 493.
Madanagopalan, N., Shiner, M. and Rowe, B. (1965), *Amer. J. Med.*, **38**, 42.
Madden, J. L., Ravid, J. M. and Haddad, J. R. (1969), *Ann. Surg.*, **170**, 351.
Meadows, T. R. and Batsakis, J. G. (1963), *Arch. Surg. Chicago*, **87**, 976.
Ming, S. C., Simon, M. and Tandon, B. N. (1963), *Gastroenterology*, **44**, 63.
Morson, B. C. and Lockhart-Mummery, H. E. (1959), *Lancet*, **2**, 1122.
Morson, B. C. (1966), *Gastroenterology*, **51**, 807.
Morson, B. C. (1968), *Proc. Roy. Soc. Med.*, **61**, 79.
Mountain, J. C. (1970), *Gut*, **11**, 18.
Parrish, R. A., Karsten, M. B., McRae, A. T. and Moretz, W. H. (1968), *Amer. J. Surg.*, **115**, 371.
Perrett, A. D., Truelove, S. C. and Massarella, G. R. (1968), *Brit. med. J.*, **2**, 466.
Pope, C. E. (1970), *Gastroenterology*, **58**, 414.
Rappaport, H., Burgoyne, F. H. and Smetana, H. F. (1951), *Mil. Surgeon*, **109**, 463.
Rippey, J. H. and Sommers, S. C. (1967), *Amer. J. Digest. Dis.*, **12**, 465.
Rodaniche, E. C., Kirsner, J. B. and Palmer, W. L. (1943), *Gastroenterology*, **1**, 687.
Schmidt, G. T., Lennard-Jones, J. E., Morson, B. C. and Young A. C. (1968), *Gut*, **9**, 7.
Schofield. P. F. (1965), *Ann. Roy. Coll. Surg. Engl.*, **36**, 258.
Sheil, F. O., Clark, C. G. and Goligher, J. C. (1968), *Brit. J. Surg.*, **55**, 53.
Shiner, M. and Drury, R. A. B. (1962), *Amer. J. Digest. Dis.*, **7**, 744.
Tyers, G. F. O., Steiger, E. and Dudrick, S. J. (1969), *Ann. Surg.*, **169**, 510.
Van der Hoeden, R., Bremer, A. and Parmentier, R. (1969), *Acta Gastroent. Belg.*, **32**, 171.
Van Patter, W. N., Bargen, J. A., Dockerty, M. B., Feldman, W. H., Mayo, C. W. and Waugh, J. M. (1954), *Gastroenterology*, **26**, 347.
Warren, S. and Sommers, S. C. (1948), *Amer. J. Path.*, **24**, 475.
Wells, C. (1952), *Ann. Roy. Coll. Surg. Engl.*, **11**, 105.
Williams, W. J. (1964), *Gut*, **5**, 510.
Wyatt, A. P. (1969), *Gut*, **10**, 924.

Chapter V
Clinical Features

Many patients with Crohn's disease have inflammation in both the small and the large intestine. The relative importance of the various signs and symptoms described in this chapter varies somewhat between the two types. Because the large intestine is now involved with increasing frequency, it is advisable to consider the clinical features of each type separately. In practice there is considerable overlap between the two disease patterns, and the subdivision is an arbitrary one.

Natural History

In nearly all cases, Crohn's disease runs a chronic relapsing course. No proven example of spontaneous cure of the chronic small intestinal form has been recorded. Follow-up studies of large bowel disease have not yet been carried on for a sufficient number of years to enable a definite statement about cure to be made. It seems improbable that bowel with chronic transmural inflammation could ever return completely to normal. The remissions and relapses in Crohn's disease mostly are less clear-cut than for example they are in ulcerative colitis or duodenal ulceration. Without surgical intervention, the course tends to be progressive, with exacerbations of symptoms superimposed on a background of gradually deteriorating health. Few unoperated patients can maintain their general condition without taking numerous drugs. Eventually 9 out of 10 patients require surgical intervention, although with the introduction of immunosuppressive agents, in the future such intervention may be postponed for a longer time than was formerly the case.

It is impossible to predict the exact clinical course that will be pursued by any new patient. Sometimes the symptoms may be relatively mild, allowing the patient to live a normal life for many months or years; additional symptoms may be slow to appear. This is unusual. More often the disease causes symptoms which soon interfere with work and pleasure. In spite of symptomatic drug treatment, new manifestations develop although the correct diagnosis may still not have been made. In the Aberdeen series of 175 patients* whose clinical course was studied in detail, there was a mean interval of 19 months between the onset of symptoms and the diagnosis being established. However, the interval

* This total includes some patients who were excluded from the epidemiological study.

varied widely and showed a very skew distribution. The median (or most common) time lapse between onset and diagnosis was only 6 months.

While between 80 and 90 per cent of cases commence insidiously and follow the progressive course outlined above (Williams, 1971) there are some patients in whom the onset is sudden and who are admitted to hospital as acute emergencies. The provisional diagnosis is usually acute appendicitis or intestinal obstruction. Eighteen Aberdeen patients fell into this category. At laparotomy there was thickening and redness of the terminal ileum; no definitive surgery was performed. Ten out of the 18 patients had no further trouble on clinical and radiological follow-up studies. They probably did not have genuine Crohn's disease (see pgs. 66, 75) and they are not included in the total of 175 patients in the Aberdeen series. Eight patients with an apparently short clinical history went on to develop other evidence of Crohn's disease in a few weeks or months. On radiological examination their lower ileum never looked normal; on more detailed interrogation 6 out of the 8 patients admitted that they had had occasional episodes of diarrhoea prior to developing the acute symptoms which had precipitated their admission. These patients are considered to be examples of the acute onset of chronic Crohn's disease.

Presentation

The complete clinical picture of a disease is formed not only by the various symptoms and signs that appear, but also by the order of their appearance and by their behaviour over a period of time. The type of patient affected and the first symptom frequently give an important clue to the correct diagnosis. The majority of patients are women, often young. They must first be questioned about the possibility of food-poisoning or other acquired forms of gastroenteritis, and about any irritants or drugs that they may have taken. The clinical features described below are based largely on the experience gained from studying the 175 patients with chronic Crohn's disease seen in north-east Scotland (Kyle 1971.)

Small Intestine

More than half of the patients with small bowel disease state that abdominal pain was their first symptom (Table 1). Usually the pain is of a colicky nature, with short-lived spasms frequently precipitated by taking food. Seven of the 82 patients said that the pain was either generalized or could appear in any part of their abdomen; 18 described it as right sided and 15 as being in the lower abdomen. In 40 patients the colicky pain was experienced in the right iliac fossa. Only 2 patients claimed that it started in the epigastrium. Pain was a slightly more

Table 1

Presentation in 175 patients with chronic Crohn's disease

Symptom	Small intestine	Large intestine
Abdominal pain	82*	9
Diarrhoea	26	18
Vomiting	6	1
Rectal bleeding	5	5
Spondylitis, arthritis	5	—
Distension, mass	2	1
Weight loss	3	—
Other	11	1
Total	140	35

* Onset was acute in 8 of these patients.

common presenting symptom in male patients than in females. Approximately 1 in 6 of all male patients with abdominal pain also noticed that they had become constipated. Colicky pain is frequently accompanied by increasingly embarrassing borborygmi.

Almost 20 per cent of all patients were troubled by diarrhoea before pain became noticeable. The number of bowel movements per 24 hours varied between 2 and 12, the commonest number being 4. Blood was not usually noticed in the initial stages; only 5 patients with small bowel disease presented with this complaint. Diarrhoea was slightly commoner in female than in male patients. A few females experienced nausea and vomiting as their first symptoms. Flatulence troubled 3 patients.

In 5 patients the initial complaint was of an orthopaedic nature. Two of these patients had ankylosing spondylitis, 2 had arthritis of major joints and one patient was referred on account of a flexion deformity of the hip. Three female patients initially were suspected of having ovarian cysts because they had noticed lower abdominal distension, or a mass. One female presented with vaginal bleeding.

Intestinal inflammation is a frequently forgotten cause of a pyrexia of unknown origin (Lee and Davies, 1961; Rakatansky, 1967). Only one Aberdeen patient presented in this way. There may be a delay of up to one year in making the correct diagnosis (Tumen, 1964). Unexplained anaemia or hypoproteinaemia rarely may be the result of Crohn's disease (Cobb, 1969). Urinary symptoms are an infrequent presentation.

Large Bowel

Sixteen out of the 35 Aberdeen patients with Crohn's disease of colon and rectum initially sought medical advice on account of diarrhoea. This mostly had been of gradual onset, and the number of bowel movements per day was considerably less than in ulcerative colitis. Two

patients did mention that in spite of their diarrhoea they did not fee
that they were getting their bowel properly evacuated. When pain wa
present first, it was usually dull in nature, localized with considerable
accuracy to the site of inflammation and often it was eased or completel
relieved by defaecation. Two patients did say that their pain wa
definitely colicky, as in small bowel disease. One patient presented witl
rectal bleeding, while several admitted that they had had haemorrhoids
for years although this latter lesion was not the reason for consulting
their doctor. A small percentage of patients may be troubled for som
years by recurrent fissures or fistula-in-ano before clear evidence of
disease in the small or large intestine appears (Morson and Lockhart-
Mummery, 1959). Since the conclusion of the main survey, one young
woman has presented with a fulminant type of colonic Crohn's disease
very closely resembling the toxic megacolon of ulcerative colitis.

Symptoms of Chronic Crohn's Disease

Small Bowel
Table 2 shows the symptoms that were present at some time in the 14C
patients with Crohn's disease before they received definitive treatment
Pain, diarrhoea and weight loss constituted the classical triad and thes
symptoms when they appear in a person in the third decade of life shoul
be regarded as very suggestive of Crohn's disease.

Table 2

*Symptoms present in 140 patients with chronic
Crohn's disease of the small intestine*

Symptom	No. of cases	Per cent
Abdominal pain	119	85
Diarrhoea	87	62
Weight loss	70	50
Vomiting	67	48
Fever	57	41
Dysuria, Frequency	38	27
Sweating	21	14
Rectal bleeding	18	13

In Aberdeen 85 per cent of patients complained of abdominal pain
in Uppsala the percentage was 100 (Krause *et al.*, 1971); in London 8
per cent had pain (Dyer and Dawson, 1970), but at the Mayo Clini
several decades ago pain was recorded in only 67 per cent (Van Patte
et al., 1954). Diarrhoea and weight loss were present in 85 and 90 pe
cent of patients respectively of the Swedish patients. These figures ar
higher than the 62 per cent and 50 per cent in north-east Scotland, an
66 per cent and 55 per cent from St Bartholomew's Hospital, London
Incidence figures recorded from the Mayo Clinic for these feature

occupy an intermediate position between the findings in Sweden and those in Britain. It must be pointed out that the authors of some of these other series did not differentiate between small and large bowel disease.

While lassitude and loss of weight are common features of Crohn's disease, they were rarely the first manifestations that sent the patients to their doctor. Malaise, lassitude and anorexia all tend to be worse during an exacerbation of the disease process. Some patients will be aware that eating precipitates abdominal colic and may voluntarily restrict their intake for this reason. Insufficient calorie intake undoubtedly contributes to the common loss of weight, and absorption of the food that is eaten may be defective. Only 4 per cent of the Aberdeen patients looked cachectic and showed multiple deficiency syndromes in spite of therapy. Untreated it is certain that gross malnutrition would have appeared very much more frequently. Four young girls had failed to grow normally, a not uncommon finding in children with Crohn's disease (see page 82). Anaemia is common in patients with chronic disease.

Fever is a variable symptom. Only 13 per cent of the Swedish patients (Krause *et al.*, 1971) had attacks of fever. Among the 600 patients at the Mayo Clinic (Van Patter *et al.*, 1954) and the 100 cases of Crohn's disease studied at the Cleveland Clinic (Daffner and Brown, 1958) fever was noted in about 33 per cent. None of these writers defined the term "fever". At some time during their illness and before they came to definitive surgery, 41 per cent of the Aberdeen patients had a temperature of 38°C (100·4°F) or higher. During most of their illness there was no pyrexia. Elevations of temperature were not uncommon in the post-operative period. Sweating is not normally regarded as a feature of Crohn's disease. It is more often associated with tuberculosis. However, 15 per cent of the Aberdeen patients specifically mentioned sweating.

Urinary symptoms were present in 27 per cent of the Aberdeen patients, and were more common in females than in males. Usually the symptom was frequency of micturition, more troublesome at night than during the day. Dysuria sometimes developed and a small number of people had pain of renal origin or suffered from strangury.

Hudson (1963) reported that at St Mark's Hospital, London, almost a quarter of the female patients had symptoms of gynaecological interest. The proportion was much lower in Aberdeen but some females did complain of vaginal discharge or dyspareunia. In most of these patients the inflamed ileum had become adherent to the tube, ovary or vault of the vagina; in some a tubo-ovarian abscess developed. Contrary to the opinion expressed by Hudson (1963) Crohn's disease did appear to affect menstruation and fertility. Of the 63 female patients who had small bowel inflammation and were in the reproductive phase of life, 19 had noticed either oligomenorrhoea or secondary amenorrhoea. Six married women had been infertile for some years before coming to definitive surgery.

Large Bowel
Diarrhoea and weight loss were more common among the Aberdeen patients than was abdominal pain (Table 3). Bleeding per rectum is seldom severe and is less frequent than in ulcerative colitis; it was reported by nearly half of the patients with colonic disease. These

Table 3

Symptoms in Crohn's disease of the colon and rectum

Symptom	No. of cases	Per cent
Diarrhoea	26	74
Weight loss	26	74
Abdominal pain	24	68
Vomiting	18	51
Rectal bleeding	17	49
Dysuria, Frequency	4	11

findings are similar to those reported by Lockhart-Mummery and Morson (1964). The majority of these patients were female, which may account for the high incidence of vomiting. Considering their relatively high average age, it is surprising that urinary difficulties were rather infrequent. Many of the older patients looked pale, but none looked cachectic. Only the 4 oldest patients complained of malaise and weakness. They appeared to have become exhausted by their diarrhoea, with its resulting fluid and electrolyte losses.

Physical Signs
The presence of a tender, elongated mass in the line of the terminal ileum or large bowel is valuable confirmatory evidence in a patient with symptoms suggestive of Crohn's disease. In practice a mass is more often absent than present. Only 40 per cent of cases with large or small bowel disease in Aberdeen had a palpable mass. At the Mayo Clinic a mass was present in 31 per cent and at St Bartholomew's Hospital, London, in only 24 per cent of patients. Gurgling sounds may be elicited when the bowel adjacent to the mass is compressed. Very occasionally a pelvic mass will first be detected on rectal examination.

Deep tenderness is noted in nearly 2 out of 3 patients, and digital examination of the rectum often causes considerable discomfort. Abdominal distension is a manifestation of subacute intestinal obstruction of chronic type. It is likely to become more prominent during exacerbations of the disease, but in some patients with scattered lesions and multiple adhesions, the abdomen always remains tumid, even during a remission. Loss of protein from the ulcerated intestine can result in oedema. Four Aberdeen patients had leg oedema extending up to knee level, and minor degrees of ankle oedema are not uncommon.

Clubbing of the finger tips and increased curvature of the nails are two other features sometimes seen in Crohn's disease. A prospective survey would be necessary to determine how often they are present. Fielding and Cooke (1971) looked at the fingers of 181 patients in Birmingham and noticed that 105 (58 per cent) showed evidence of clubbing. There was increase in the volume of the pulp, greater curvature of the nail and hyperaemia, particularly at the nail fold which may almost resemble a chronic paronychia. Changes in the finger tips reflect the activity of the disease in the intestine. Within a few weeks from the start of a remission, spontaneous or drug-induced, a new, smoother and more uniform nail can be seen emerging.

The reported incidence of perianal lesions varies greatly. Fissures and fistulae, large shallow ulcers, haemorrhoids and skin tags may be present, but it would appear that only a very small proportion of the patients who have them ever complain about them. With careful inspection of the anal canal and perianal skin, Fielding (1969) believed that some lesion would be found in 3 out of 4 patients, mostly consisting of either bluish oedematous skin tags or a painless posterior fissure (Fig. 1). The severity of the patient's diarrhoea affects the size of the skin tags. All perianal lesions are more common when the granulomatous disease is present in the distal large bowel. Fielding stated that over 90 per cent of cases with *colonic* Crohn's disease had these lesions. Such a high percentage has not been observed by others. It is only likely to be recorded when patients have had the disease, and have been followed, for a considerable number of years, the perianal region and anal canal being carefully inspected at each hospital attendance. One difficulty in the interpretation of the figures relating to perianal lesions is the rarity of control series properly matched for age and sex. Fielding (1969) considered the incidence in colonic Crohn's disease to be more than double that for control subjects.

While progression of ileal Crohn's disease proximally (or distally) is usually slow, taking many months or years, in the colon the disease may spread very much more rapidly.

"Acute Regional Ileitis"

Reference has already been made (page 70) to the acute onset of inflammatory disease in the small intestine. In approximately one case in 10 the patient's symptoms have only been present for a few hours or days; a small number admit to having had slight diarrhoea earlier, before acute pain started. Compared to acute appendicitis, vomiting may be less common in patients with ileal inflammation, and no rebound sign may be elicited. Pyrexia is likely to be more marked than in moderately severe Crohn's disease and 50 per cent or more of the patients are males.

After being followed up for months or years, and having had radiological studies, 10 out of the 18 Aberdeen patients (55 per cent) were considered not to have Crohn's disease. At the Mount Sinai Hospital,

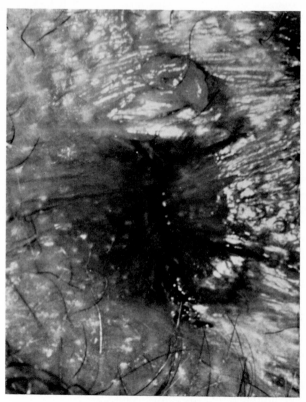

Fig. 1. Painless posterior fissure and an anterior skin tag in a patient with Crohn's disease of ileum.

New York, 57 per cent of so-called "acute regional ileitis" patients did not progress to chronic granulomatous disease. Examination of 9 resected specimens showed an acute suppurative reaction and no histological characteristics of Crohn's disease. Free perforation had occurred in a few patients. More than 90 per cent of the patients seen by Gump *et al.* (1967) with acute ileitis at the Presbyterian Hospital, New York, remained completely free of any evidence of recurrent intestinal disease for an average of 9 years.

It seems clear that there are numerous different diseases, resembling each other in their symptomatology and to a lesser extent in their macroscopic appearance, that are being grouped together as acute ileitis. This is unfortunate, but with the present lack of knowledge about aetiology it is probably unavoidable. It is known that inflammation may be visible on the serosal aspect of the ileum in mesenteric adenitis (Busson and Bard, 1960). There were some cases of ileitis among British troops with enteric infection in Egypt (Cowan, 1958); these did not go on to develop chronic symptoms. The ileum may look inflamed in typhoid fever (Bosseckert, 1965). Other agents may be responsible for very acute, self-limiting inflammation in the jejunum.

The majority of emergency operations for suspected appendicitis in Britain are performed by comparatively junior and inexperienced members of the surgical staff. On reviewing the 10 Aberdeen patients initially labelled as acute Crohn's disease, it was obvious that the young operator had had little or no opportunity of seeing genuine Crohn's disease. One of the patients had had a mesenteric infarct and required a resection 48 hours after the first laparotomy. Another patient had round-worm infestation. Misdiagnosis by the inexperienced probably accounts for a sizeable part of any series of patients thought to have acute ileitis. In the remainder some viral, bacterial or parasitic agent is probably responsible and the condition is not related to chronic Crohn's disease.

There may be no clinical test or investigation available in the emergency situation that will enable the doctor to separate patients with acute right lower abdominal pain into different aetiological groups. If the symptoms and signs are such as to give ground for believing that the patient may have acute suppurative appendicitis or peritonitis, then laparotomy is mandatory. The life-threatening lesion can be dealt with at operation or the erroneous diagnosis be refuted, but in the latter circumstance the exact nature of the intestinal lesion may still be in doubt. Very rarely Crohn's disease is initially confined to the appendix (Ewen *et al.*, 1970) and only manifests itself elsewhere in the intestinal tract at a later date.

Cutaneous Lesions in Crohn's Disease

For many years Crohn's disease was regarded as a condition only encountered in the columnar epithelium of the intestinal tract. Recently, as large series have been studied in greater detail, it has been realized that typical granulomatous lesions may be found in squamous epithelium. The indolent ulcers and fissures in and extending from the anal canal are now well known. External fistulae onto the abdominal wall are increasingly rare in Aberdeen and no persistent ulceration related to such fistulae has been seen by the author. However, this type of ulceration sometimes occurs. With severe and protracted disease, particularly of the distal colon and rectum, there may be long linear ulcers in the perineum, extending forwards into the labia in the female or alongside the scrotum towards the base of the penis in the males. Rarely there are multiple ulcers, separate from each other and from the anal margin. A shallow ulcer may appear beneath the breast, around the umbilicus or below a fold of skin on the abdomen (Mountain, 1970); histological examination of a biopsy specimen may reveal typical changes of Crohn's disease. It must be emphasized that except in the perianal region these ectopic ulcers are very rare.

Crohn's Disease of the Mouth

Aphthous ulceration is a painful and unpredictable complication in some patients with intestinal Crohn's disease. About 20 per cent of patients have this type of ulceration at some stage during their illness. Sometimes it is more marked or first appears during a severe exacerbation or immediately after an abdominal operation. At such times there is an understandable reluctance to add to the patient's discomfort by performing biopsies on oral lesions. Crohn's disease may appear in the mouth (Dudeney, 1969) and it seems probable that if more of the aphthous ulcers were studied under the microscope, a higher incidence of granulomatous lesions within the mouth would be found. Schiller *et al.* (1971) have described 6 patients with ulcers or polypoid masses within the mouth or fissures on the lips, biopsies showing changes compatible with Crohn's disease. Five of the patients had known intestinal disease. In the sixth, radiological study has so far failed to demonstrate any abnormality in the gastro-intestinal tract. One recent case in Aberdeen may fall into the latter category, where an oral lesion precedes intestinal symptoms.

Oesophageal Stricture and Crohn's Disease

If typical granulomatous lesions can appear in the squamous mucosa of the mouth there would not appear to be any fundamental reason why a similar abnormality should not arise in the oesophagus. However, the concept of Crohn's disease of the oesophagus has not found ready acceptance. Dyer *et al.* (1969) reviewed 12 of the largest series of Crohn's disease that have been published and among more than 2,500 patients there was not a single example of oesophageal involvement. Nevertheless, in their own series of 198 patients these investigators had 2 patients with probable granulomatous lesions in the lower oesophagus. Pathognomonic histological changes were not present in the first case but were present in the second man, who had had an ileal resection for Crohn's disease. Dyer and his associates did not think the stricture could have resulted from prolonged nasogastric intubation. In 1968, Gelfand and Krone reported a man who developed dysphagia 3 months after the onset of colonic Crohn's disease. Endoscopy showed hyperaemia and oedema; an ulcer in mid-oesophagus responded to high doses of prednisone. Biopsy in this patient revealed non-specific oesophagitis, so that a direct association with his Crohn's disease is not certain, although the therapeutic response suggests that the two lesions were connected in some way. Madden *et al.* (1969) have also described a condition in the oesophagus simulating Crohn's disease.

Gastroduodenal Involvement in Crohn's Disease

It has been known for over 20 years that the stomach and duodenum might be involved in the granulomatous process of Crohn's disease (Comfort *et al.*, 1950). The condition appeared to be rare, or was rarely recognized. Several large series, such as that from the Mayo Clinic (Van Patter *et al.*, 1954) did not include any examples. However, during the last few years there have been several reports and reviews on the subject (Johnson *et al.*, 1966; Burgess *et al.*, 1971; Wise *et al.*, 1971). The incidence of abnormalities in the stomach and duodenum may be as high as 4 per cent—12 cases among the 300 patients in the Birmingham region (Fielding *et al.*, 1970).

In some patients upper abdominal symptoms only start months or years after Crohn's disease has been detected lower down the alimentary tract. Rather more frequently some distortion of stomach and duodenum is noted by the radiologist during a barium examination requested for more obviously intestinal complaints such as diarrhoea. The finding may be regarded as incidental, the result of old peptic ulceration, but in the future more detailed study by endoscopy and biopsy may reveal that the underlying disease process is granulomatous.

Pain in the epigastrium is the most common symptom, and may mimic duodenal ulceration. Eating food often makes the pain worse; alkalis give temporary relief in many instances. When there is narrowing of the pylorus, infiltration in the gastric wall or distortion of the duodenum, nausea and vomiting are likely to be troublesome. The vomiting may resemble that of pyloric stenosis, with very large gastric residues suddenly being vomited during the night or early morning. Weight loss is inevitable, and a gastric succussion splash may readily be elicited. Approximately half the patients have episodic diarrhoea. Endoscopy may show bizarre distortions or proliferative lesions particularly in the vicinity of the gastric antrum and pylorus. The surface may be ulcerated. Several biopsy specimens are often needed before a confident diagnosis can be made.

Only one young man has had Crohn's disease in the gastric antrum and duodenum in the Aberdeen series of 175 patients. He had had epigastric pain for 2 years and the radiological appearances had been interpreted as scarring from duodenal ulceration. Then he developed frank colonic symptoms, with diarrhoea and lower abdominal pain and eventually he required a hemicolectomy. During this operation biopsies were taken from the gastro-duodenal region and confirmed the presence of granulomatous disease there. Skip lesions were present in the small intestine.

When the duodenum at and close to the papilla of the pancreatic duct is involved there are likely to be recurrent attacks of pancreatitis (Hoffman *et al.*, 1971), presumably from duct obstruction.

Crohn's Disease Confined to the Jejunum

Only a very small percentage of patients have the disease confined to the upper small intestine. Much more frequently jejunal involvement appears as a proximal extension of disease in the distal ileum, although the lesions may have arisen simultaneously. Vomiting is a prominent feature of Crohn's disease in the jejunum, and there is often hypoproteinaemia, with oedema. Some patients have a protein-losing enteropathy (Moynagh, 1968) and on inspection of resected specimens there is very extensive ulceration of the mucosal surface. Diverticula of the jejunum are present in many cases and may result from the narrowing of the lumen that the granulomatous process produces. Bacterial proliferation within the diverticulae produced a megaloblastic anaemia and other deficiencies in 2 Aberdeen patients.

Crohn's Disease of the Rectum

Many patients with Crohn's disease of the colon also have the disease in the rectum (Deucher and Widmer, 1970). The cobblestone, ulcerated and rather rigid and oedematous state of the rectal mucosa is obvious on sigmoidoscopy (Crohn, 1960; Rudell *et al.*, 1968). The less usual and more worrying group of patients are those in whom the rectal lesion simulates a neoplasm or stricture. Often they are old: 3 out of the 8 patients with major rectal lesions seen in Aberdeen were over 70 years and a patient from South Africa was 82 years old (Brom *et al.*, 1968). Two of the Scottish patients presented with what looked like an anal epithelioma, although the surrounding skin was rather more bluish than is usually seen with an ordinary neoplasm. In 2 patients on digital examination there seemed to be a long, irregular carcinoma encircling most of the rectal wall. Three patients presented initially with what on sigmoidoscopy and biopsy seemed to be a mild, localized proctitis. They rapidly reappeared after a course of conventional therapy, with weight loss, diarrhoea and the passage of blood per rectum. It was immediately feared that a rectal cancer had been missed at the first examination. The rectal lumen was very distorted and could not be distended by insufflating air through the sigmoidoscope. Numerous biopsy specimens showed granulomas and giant cells. Many patients with rectal disease do have fistulae and ulcers in the perianal skin, and there may be large, flat ulcers in the anal canal and lower rectum.

Pregnancy and Crohn's Disease

Crohn's disease causes less trouble in pregnancy than might be anticipated. Any form of intraperitoneal inflammation is worrying when the
patient is pregnant. Pain commencing on the right side may be wrongly
diagnosed as urinary infection, appendicitis, a ruptured tubal pregnancy, or spontaneous abortion. Females with Crohn's disease may
have some difficulty in becoming pregnant. Nearly one-third of the
married female patients in the Birmingham series apparently were
infertile (Fielding and Cooke, 1970); patients with Crohn's disease of
the colon were less fertile than those with ileal disease. Crohn *et al.*
(1956) at Mount Sinai Hospital noted that 32 out of 85 married females
had no children. During the 15 years of the Aberdeen survey there were
63 females between the ages of 17 years and 47 years. Approximately
two-thirds of this total were married. However, an infertility incidence
cannot be calculated directly from these figures. Most married women
bear children during their twenties and early thirties, a few may not
want children, and there may be other reasons for family limitation. It
is known that in Aberdeen 6 females had been extensively investigated
for infertility for some years before receiving effective treatment for
their bowel disease. Failure to conceive is not necessarily the result of
tubal occlusion by inflammation. Inadequate uptake of vitamin B_{12} or
other essential factor and the poor state of the patient's general health
may be important. Conception may take place rapidly after resection of
chronically inflamed terminal ileum, although no procedure has been
carried out on the Fallopian tubes.

It is unusual for Crohn's disease to be present for the first time
during pregnancy. When Blair and Allen (1962) described their young
lady they could find only 6 comparable cases in the literature. The
bowel symptoms had usually appeared during the 6th or 7th month of
pregnancy and several patients went into premature labour. Two babies
and one mother died. When a patient with known Crohn's disease
became pregnant, Fielding and Cooke (1970) found no increase in the
risk of abortion, prematurity, still-birth or of congenital abnormalities.
Schofield *et al.* (1970) had a less happy experience, the above cited
complications developing in one-third of pregnancies, particularly when
Crohn's disease was located in the colon. The author has supervised
numerous young female patients during pregnancy without encounter-
ing any untoward difficulties in the mother or abnormalities in the child.
Heyworth *et al.* (1970) had to deal with large intra-abdominal abscesses
in 2 of their pregnant patients.

Having remained in fair or even improved general health during
pregnancy, between 25 and 40 per cent of the Birmingham patients had
an exacerbation of their intestinal disease during the puerperium. This
experience is at variance with that in Aberdeen where the only difficulty
has been to persuade mothers with new babies to attend the Follow Up

Clinic. No patient in Aberdeen has been specifically advised to avoid pregnancy; several have had tubal ligation performed after producing 2 or 3 healthy children.

Crohn's Disease in Children

Very young children do not appear to show evidence of active Crohn's disease, although Koop *et al.* (1947) did describe one case of "cicatrizing enterocolitis" in a neonate. True Crohn's disease is rare before 10 years of age. In the Aberdeen (epidemiology) series of 166 patients there was no definite case that had started during the first decade. One patient did give a doubtful history of "a tendency to diarrhoea all his life", but abdominal colic did not commence until he was almost 15 years old. Eight patients first noticed symptoms between 10 and 15 years; 4 were boys and 4 girls, a higher proportion of males than that noted among adult patients (page 19). Male preponderance is even more marked in Sweden. Ten of the 13 cases reported frum Lund were males (Hansing and Meeuwisse, 1971) and there were 24 boys among 36 patients seen at the Karolinska Sjukhuset in Stockholm (Ehrenpreis *et al.*, 1971). In the United States, Silverman (1966) saw 8 boys and 6 girls with Crohn's disease in Cincinnatti, while at the Mayo Clinic there were 42 boys and 13 girls (van Heerden *et al.*, 1967). Experience in the Swedish capital suggests that there has been a considerable increase in the incidence of Crohn's disease in children since 1959.

As in adults, the commonest presenting symptoms are colicky abdominal pain and diarrhoea. Rectal bleeding is less frequent than in ulcerative colitis. When the history is very short the child may be thought to have acute appendicitis. With a longer history of recurrent lower abdominal pain an atypical or retrocaecal appendicitis may be suspected and laparotomy undertaken. Sometimes there is a history of recurrent perianal abscesses and fissures; these always merit full investigation in children. The diagnosis is liable to be delayed when symptoms are general rather than local. The onset to diagnosis interval exceeded 4 years in 7 out of the 36 Stockholm children. These 7 young patients were first seen on account of retardation of growth (McCaffrey, 1970), delayed menarche and recurrent lassitude and pyrexia of unknown origin. Ehrenpreis *et al.* (1971) have provided a striking picture of 13-year-old identical twins, one having Crohn's disease and being almost a head shorter than her sister. Weight loss is universal, anorexia common and faecal protein loss may be severe, so it is not surprising that growth is arrested. Some of these children initially have been referred to endocrinologists, while others have had psychiatric treatment for suspected anorexia nervosa. The addition of Crohn's disease to the group of conditions requiring differential diagnosis in patients failing to grow will permit earlier diagnosis. Symptoms indicating gastro-intestinal disease may be late in appearing. An occasional child presents with erythema nodosum or with persistently raised erythrocyte sedimentation rate (ESR) or serum gammaglobulin level (Hansing and Meeuwisse, 1971) but sooner or later abdominal pain and diarrhoea develop in every young patient.

Nearly all children with Crohn's disease have iron-deficiency anaemia. Clubbing of the fingers and oedema of the ankles are present in 15 per cent. A palpable abdominal mass is less common than in adults. A right lower abdominal mass was felt in only 4 out of the 36 Stockholm children. Colonic involvement is more frequent than in older patients and this may partly account for the absence of a palpable abnormality in the region of the terminal ileum. Arthritic symptoms are occasionally present, and may erroneously be attributed to rheumatoid arthritis. Paediatricians should be more aware of intestinal disease being the cause for unexplained growth retardation, menstrual irregularities, skin and joint symptoms. Careful radiological examination in a department experienced in paediatric work is needed to detect the changes produced by Crohn's disease in the child's distal small intestine.

Associated Diseases

The distinction between what may be termed associated diseases and those conditions that may be regarded as complications of Crohn's disease is admittedly artificial. In this chapter duodenal ulceration, asthma and hay fever and a variety of skin lesions are considered as associated diseases, for many of them antedate the onset of Crohn's disease in the intestine. However, the more serious types of dermatological disease generally only appear during exacerbations of the intestinal inflammation, and in that sense they are complications.

Duodenal Ulceration

The exact incidence is not known. It must be remembered that those who suffer from Crohn's disease are subjected to very many more radiological investigations than are healthy members of the population. An occasional slight abnormality seen on one out of a great many films may be misinterpreted as being the result of ulceration. The possibility that some of these abnormalities are in fact accounted for by gastroduodenal Crohn's disease is mentioned above. Freud and Spellberg (1957) had 10 male patients with ulcers out of 43 patients with proven Crohn's disease, an incidence of 23 per cent. Because 5 of the men developed epigastric pain after treatment for their Crohn's disease had begun, the writers were concerned about the possible role of corticosteroids in the causation of the ulcers. At the Lahey Clinic, Boston, between 1963 and 1969 the incidence of duodenal ulceration was 10·3 per cent among 117 patients with Crohn's disease (Latchis *et al.*, 1971). In Birmingham, since 1944, the incidence has been 8 per cent (Fielding and Cooke, 1970). This is a relatively high figure considering that in

Britain Crohn's disease is rather more common in females, not more than 2 per cent of whom would be expected to have an ulcer during middle life. Twelve out of the 175 Aberdeen patients at some time have been diagnosed as having a duodenal ulcer. In at least 3 of them there is reason for thinking that the duodenal deformity may have resulted from adhesions or granulomatous disease.

Fielding and Cooke (1970) mention the increase in gastric acid output that often follows intestinal resection, and suggest that this hyper-secretion may account for some of the ulcers that appear in advanced and recurrent disease. In the absence of any radiologically studied control population, it is not possible to state if the incidence of duodenal ulceration in untreated and uncomplicated Crohn's disease is unusually high. Therapy renders any postulated association even more difficult to unravel.

Asthma and Hay Fever (*Allergic Rhinitis*)

The names of both these allergic conditions are frequently misused, and even with careful explanation and interrogation patients often give misleading information. Chronic bronchitis may be called asthma and a common cold be referred to as the rather popular diagnosis of hay fever. These difficulties and sources of error must be borne in mind when considering figures concerning the incidence of the two conditions in Crohn's disease. Hammer and her colleagues (1968) in Bristol carried out the most accurate survey. The prevalence of asthma among the 45 Crohn's patients interviewed was 4 per cent. In the control series of 319 people, 3 per cent said they had asthma so that there was no difference between the groups. However, 18 per cent of patients were considered to have allergic rhinitis compared to 6 per cent of the general hospital population. This difference is statistically significant. Furthermore, allergic rhinitis was more prevalent in the relatives of patients than in the relatives of control subjects.

Skin Lesions

The most comprehensive study of dermatological abnormalities in Crohn's disease is that carried out by McCallum and Kinmont (1968). They questioned numerous clinicians, and reported that skin lesions were present in no less than 43 per cent of patients with Crohn's disease. Unfortunately they included fistulae in the perianal zone (17 per cent) and abdominal wall (20 per cent). Such fistulae are known to be com-mon; the incidence of genuine dermatological conditions in the survey is 6 per cent. This percentage refers to conditions present at the time that the patient was under treatment for intestinal disease. An associated disease may be present beforehand. Forty out of the 175 Aberdeen patients stated that they had had skin trouble at some time in their lives. This incidence is in close agreement with that noted at St Bartholomew's Hospital, London (Dyer *et al.*, 1970). Thirty-two said they had had eczema. This is almost certainly an underestimate. It is difficult for adults to remember all the diseases they may have had in childhood. Furthermore the accuracy of the diagnosis often was doubtful. It was noticeable that many of the patients when directly questioned were much more certain about their own children having eczema. After interviewing 45 patients with Crohn's disease, Hammer *et al.* (1968) recorded an incidence of eczema of 33 per cent compared to 7 per cent in the control population, the difference being highly significant. Among first degree relatives the incidence was lower than in the propositi, but the relatives included parents and siblings as well as children.

The next most common skin lesion after eczema in patients with Crohn's disease is erythema nodosum (Jacobs, 1959). Six of the Aberdeen patients had the raised, red, irregular skin lesions on legs or arms, often appearing or becoming more florid during an active phase of the intestinal disease. Two patients were receiving treatment for psoriasis. Pyoderma gangrenosum, well recognized in ulcerative colitis, is very rare in Crohn's disease (Stathers, 1967); cutaneous polyarteritis nodosa around the ankles has also been described (Dyer *et al.*, 1970). No example of either condition has been seen in north-east Scotland.

When confronted by an unusual skin rash in a patient with a progressive and unpredictable disease, the clinician must always remember the possibility of the rash being the result of a drug reaction.

References

Blair, J. S. G. and Allen, N. (1962), *J. Obstet. Gynec. Br. Comm.*, **69**, 648.
Bosseckert, H. (1965), *Deutsch Z. Verd. Stoffwsc.*, **24**, 203.
Brom, B., Bank, S., Marks, I. N., Barbezat, G. and Raynham, B. (1968), *S. Afr. med. J.*, **42**, 1099.
Burgess, J. N., Legge, D. A. and Judd, E. S. (1971), *Surg. Gynec. Obstet.*, **132**, 628.
Busson, A. and Bard, M. (1960), *Arch. Dis. Appar. Dig.*, **49**, 236.
Cobb, T. C. (1969), *J.A.M.A.*, **207**, 1351.
Comfort, M. W., Weber, H. M., Baggenstoss, A. H. and Kiely, W. F. (1950), *Amer. J. med. Sci.*, **220**, 616.
Cowan, D. J. (1958), *Brit. med. J.*, **1**, 438.
Crohn, B. B., Yarnis, H. and Korelitz, B. (1956), *Gastroenterology*, **31**, 615.
Crohn, B. B. (1960), *Dis. Colon Rectum*, **3**, 99.
Crohn, B. B. (1965), *New York State J. Med.*, **65**, 641.
Daffner, J. E. and Brown, C. H. (1958), *Ann. Int. Med.*, **49**, 580.
Deucher, F. and Widmer, A. (1970), *Langenbeck Arch. Chir.*, **328**, 8.
Dudeney, T. P. (1969), *Proc. Roy. Soc. Med.*, **62**, 1237.
Dyer, N. H., Cook, P. L. and Harper, R. A. K. (1969), *Gut*, **10**, 549.
Dyer, N. H. and Dawson, A. M. (1970), *Brit. med. J.*, **1**, 735.
Dyer, N. H., Verbov, J. L., Dawson, A. M. and Borrie, P. F. (1970), *Lancet*, **1**, 648.
Ehrenpreis, T., Gierup, J. and Lagercrantz, R. (1971), *Acta Paediat. Scand.*, **60**, 209.
Ewen, S. W. B., Anderson, J., Galloway, J. M.D., Miller, J. B. and Kyle, J. (1971), *Gastroenterology*, **60**, 853.

Fielding, J. F. (1969), *Regional Enteritis*, M.D. Thesis. National University of Ireland (Cork).

Fielding, J. F. and Cooke, W. T. (1970), *Gut*, **11**, 998.

Fielding, J. F., Toye, D. K. M., Beton, D. C. and Cooke, W. T. (1970), *Gut*, **11**, 1001.

Fielding, J. F. and Cooke, W. T. (1970), *Brit. med. J.*, **2**, 76.

Fielding, J. F. and Cooke, W. T. (1971), *Gut*, **12**, 442.

Freud, W. I. and Spellberg, M. A. (1957), *Amer. J. Gastroenterol.*, **28**, 418.

Gelfand, M. D. and Krone, C. L. (1968), *Gastroenterology*, **55**, 510.

Gump, F. E., Lepore, M. and Barker, H. G. (1967), *Ann. Surg.*, **166**, 942.

Hammer, R., Ashurst, P. and Naish, J. (1968), *Gut*, **9**, 17.

Hansing, B. and Meeuwisse, G. (1971), *Acta Paediat. Scand.*, **60**, 104.

van Heerden, J. A., Sigler, R. M. and Lynn, H. B. (1967), *Proc. Mayo Clin.*, **42**, 100.

Heyworth, B., Basu, S. and Clegg, J. (1970), *Brit. Med. J.*, **2**, 363.

Hoffman, H. N., Legge, D. A. and Carlson, H. (1971), *Gastroenterology*, **60**, 676.

Hudson, C. N. (1963), *J. Obstet. Gynec. Br. Comm.*, **70**, 437.

Jacobs, W. H. (1959), *Gastroenterology*, **37**, 286.

Johnson, O. A., Hoskins, D. W., Todd, J. and Thorbjarnson, B. (1966), *Gastroenterology*, **50**, 571.

Koop, C. E., Perlingiero, J. G. and Weiss, W. (1947), *Amer. J. med. Sci.*, **214**, 27.

Krause, U., Bergman, L. and Norlen, B. J. (1971), *Scand. J. Gastroent.*, **6**, 97.

Kyle, J. (1971), *Scot. Med. J.*, **16**, 197.

Kyle, J., Cole, T. P. and Ewen, S. W. R. (1969), *Prensa med. Argent.*, **56**, 470.

Latchis, K. S., Rao, C. S. and Colcock, B. P. (1971), *Amer. J. Surg.*, **121**, 418.

Lee, F. I. and Davies, D. M. (1961), *Lancet*, **1**, 1205.

Lockhart-Mummery, H. E. and Morson, B. C. (1964), *Gut*, **5**, 493.

McCaffrey, T. D. (1970), *Pediatrics*, **45**, 386.

McCallum, D. I. and Kinmont, P. D. C. (1968), *Brit. J. Dermat.*, **80**, 1.

Madden, J. L., Ravid, J. M. and Haddad, J. R. (1969), *Ann. Surg.*, **170**, 351.

Morson, B. C. and Lockhart-Mummery, H. E. (1959), *Lancet*, **2**, 1122.

Mountain, J. C. (1970), *Gut*, **11**, 18.

Moynagh, P. D. (1968), *Proc. Roy. Soc. Med.*, **61**, 443.

Rakatansky, H. (1967), *Arch. Int. Med.*, **119**, 321.

Rudell, M., Gontier, F. and Smadja, A. (1968), *Mem. Acad. Chir. (Paris)*, **94**, 683.

Schiller, K. F. R., Golding, P. L., Peebles, R. A. and Whitehead, R. A. (1971), *Gut*, **12**, 1001.

Schofield, P. F., Turnbull, R. B. and Hawk, W. A. (1970), *Brit. med. J.*, **2**, 364.

Silverman, F. N. (1966), *Aust. Paediat. J.*, **2**, 207.

Stathers, G. M. (1967), *Arch. Dermat. (Chicago)*, **95**, 365.

Tumen, H. J. (1964), *Amer. J. Digest. Dis.*, **9**, 314.

Van Patter, W. N., Bargen, J. A., Dockerty, M., Feldman, W. H., Mayo, C. W. and Waugh, H. M. (1954), *Gastroenterology*, **26**, 350.

Williams, J. A. (1971), *Gut*, **12**, 739.

Wise, L., Kyriakos, M., McCown, A. and Ballinger, W. F. (1971), *Amer. J. Surg.*, **121**, 184.

Chapter VI
Investigation and Differential Diagnosis

The correct diagnosis of Crohn's disease should be made as quickly as possible. Too often in the past there has been considerable delay between the time the patient first noticed symptoms and the start of appropriate treatment. With greater awareness of the disease the onset to diagnosis interval should be shortened considerably, with consequent benefit to the patient and reduction in the number of unhelpful investigations that are undertaken. For acute onset, see page 75.

From the point of view of diagnosis, patients with chronic Crohn's disease fall into three groups. First, there are those presenting with the characteristic triad of colicky abdominal pain, diarrhoea and weight loss. Many of these patients will be young women in the third decade of life. In them the diagnosis should be suspected right from the beginning, and appropriate investigations to confirm the presence of granulomatous intestinal disease should be ordered. It is this first group that the proportion of rapidly made and accurate diagnoses should increase in the future.

The second and rather smaller group of patients are those who initially complain of one or two gastrointestinal symptoms, but who have not got the typical triad of Crohn's disease. Some of the findings on examination, such as a palpable, tender mass, ought to raise the possibility of Crohn's disease being responsible. More often it will be the investigations—particularly the barium enema or barium meal and follow through—that reveal the true cause of their symptoms. However, even in this group there can be little justification for delay in arriving at the correct diagnosis, provided that the patient has consulted her doctor at an early date. This is a major proviso. The onset of Crohn's disease often is insidious, and the diarrhoea is little more than a nuisance which housewives will tolerate for many months before seeking medical advice.

The third and smallest group is the one in which diagnosis is most difficult. This group consists of those patients—less than 10 per cent of the total—in whom the initial symptoms are not obviously related to the intestinal tract. Some of the women may quite correctly have been referred by their family doctor to a gynaecologist because of vaginal discharge or dyspareunia. Others may attend orthopaedic clinics on account of obscure spinal or joint pains. A few patients will puzzle a physician or haematologist with unexplained and persistent fever or anaemia. The diagnosis is finally made by a lengthy process of exclusion.

Many body systems are likely to have been studied repeatedly and in great detail, and much time may have been lost before it is realized that Crohn's disease is responsible for the symptoms. Apart from making colleagues in other specialities aware of the protean manifestations of Crohn's disease, it is difficult to see how making the diagnosis can be expedited in this third group.

Order of Investigations

Many of the investigations for Crohn's disease can be performed on an out-patient basis. When the level of clinical suspicion is high their number can often be kept small. The following 5 investigations are usually sufficient to enable the diagnosis of Crohn's disease to be made—

(i) Haematology—haemoglobin (Hb), white cell count (WBC), film and the erythrocyte sedimentation rate (ESR).
(ii) Faecal occult blood.
(iii) Blood electrolytes—sodium, potassium and urea.
(iv) Sigmoidoscopy and rectal biopsy.
(v) Radiology—barium enema, as an out-patient, followed if need be by a barium meal and follow through examination.

In most cases the provisional diagnosis will be confirmed by the result of the radiological studies. At this time medical treatment may be started, provided that the patient's general condition is clearly good and the disease is of short duration.

However, it is often desirable to obtain a better understanding of the patient's metabolic status before therapy commences, in which case the patient is admitted to hospital for a few days. Absorption and excretion tests of fat, xylose, vitamin B_{12} and calcium are performed. The results of plasma protein, immunoglobulin, serum folate and liver function tests often take several days before they come back from the laboratory. Sometimes the radiologist will suggest a few days of in-patient intensive bowel preparation before repeating a barium enema, or he may wish to carry out selective angiography. When the patient is in hospital the opportunity may be taken to perform skin tests, for example Mantoux, Kveim and Frei tests. The specificity of some of these reactions is now in considerable doubt (see pages 34 and 38). Strongly positive reactions may point towards a completely different diagnosis, but the tests themselves are of little direct help in making the diagnosis of Crohn's disease.

Bed rest in hospital plays a useful part in the non-operative treatment of Crohn's disease and especially in the minority of cases who have severe and extensive or recurrent lesions. These are the patients who are likely to show gross malabsorption and deficiency phenomena and who develop complications. Repeat absorption and balance studies are helpful in planning replacement therapy and in attempting to improve their nutritional status. Small intestinal biopsy can be of value in demonstrating the proximal extent of the Crohn's disease. Colonoscopy is sometimes of help in assessing the rate of the colon. If external fistulae have appeared fistulography can demonstrate their internal ramifications and connections. With advanced disease liver damage is liable to occur (page 131); if a biopsy has not been taken at operation then a percutaneous needle biopsy may be valuable.

It must be emphasized once again that only a small proportion of patients with Crohn's disease nowadays become severely cachectic, with multiple deficiencies, fistulae, etc. in the first months of their illness. Every patient in the Aberdeen series has been admitted to hospital at some stage in the disease. In most instances this was for routine pre-operative assessment and definitive surgery. Admission was seldom for investigation alone.

The investigations commonly performed in Crohn's disease are now considered in more detail.

Radiology

The proper radiological investigation of a patient suspected of having Crohn's disease requires careful planning. The clinician must provide the radiologist with as much pertinent information as possible, particularly in regard to details of previous abdominal operations and the signs found on examination. The majority of the patients are young and many are females, potential mothers. Watch must be kept on the total dose of irradiation that the patient receives, both during the period when the diagnosis is first being made and in later years. The natural history of confirmed Crohn's disease may extend over the greater part of the patient's life. With established disease often there is poor correlation between the radiological appearances and the clinical status; marked changes may be demonstrated in a patient who looks and feels well. Therefore it is not justifiable to order repeat barium studies simply to see how the patient is getting on. Repeat examinations should only be undertaken for some clearly defined reason, to obtain information that cannot be obtained by any other means. There is some risk of precipitating acute intestinal obstruction by giving barium to a patient who already may be sub-acutely obstructed.

Techniques

The three following methods are those commonly employed to investigate patients with Crohn's disease. An experienced radiologist will achieve a high percentage of correct diagnoses using them.

(1) *Straight Film* (*Erect and Supine*)

These films should always be examined first, before proceeding to barium studies. In many patients they will reveal evidence of sub-acute obstruction in the distal small intestine. While the site of the lesion can be determined with some accuracy, it is not possible to diagnose its cause.

In a small number of cases the straight films will reveal evidence of complications of Crohn's disease. An abscess may give rise to a soft tissue shadow, displacing loops of small intestine. Toxic megacolon is rare but immediately obvious. Examination of the sacroiliac joints may show the sclerosis caused by ankylosing spondylitis. Opaque gall-stones are sometimes seen; renal calculi are very uncommon. Free perforation into the peritoneal cavity is rare and usually gives free gas below the diaphragm. Careful examination of films would be necessary to reveal either gas in the urinary tract from a fistula or the blurring of the psoas muscle's outline that a fistula entering its sheath might cause.

(2) *Barium Enema*

In Aberdeen, a conventional barium enema is the first special radio-logical examination to be carried out. The hydrostatic pressure can be used to distend the caecum; the radiologist can evaluate the pliability of its wall and note if any spasm is present. Screening of the ileo-caecal region is most valuable. If reflux into the terminal ileum takes place good definition is obtained; the ileum is not obscured by more proximal loops of barium-filled small intestine. The sigmoid colon can overlie the ileum, but in some of these cases there will be evidence of contact spread to the sigmoid loop. After evacuation, the sigmoid mostly retracts towards the left, uncovering the lower ileum. It is at this stage of the examination that the early mucosal changes are best demonstrated. Normally reflux back through the ileo-caecal valve occurs in little more than 50 per cent of subjects. Failure to obtain reflux should arouse suspicion, and indicate the need for a barium meal and follow through examination. One of the commonest errors in the diagnosis of Crohn's disease is to accept as proof of a patient's normality a set of barium enema films which show a normal colon but which fail to outline the ileum.

Some radiologists prefer the air contrast type of enema. It is a useful technique for showing up intraluminal projections such as pseudo-polypi. Contractibility of the wall cannot be assessed by it, early mucosal changes may be effaced and fine granularity in the recto-sigmoid is hard to interpret. However, the personal preference and the experience of the radiologist with any given technique are important factors in determining its usefulness in making an accurate diagnosis.

At St Mark's Hospital, London, an "instant enema" is used routinely for patients with inflammatory bowel disease. After taking a plain film to exclude toxic dilatation, some micropaque is run into the unprepared bowel. If inflammatory disease is present the colon will be empty, and good films will usually be obtained (Lennard-Jones, 1971).

(3) *Barium Meal and Follow Through*
Raybar, a non-flocculating barium preparation, is the contrast medium commonly employed. Its passage into the distal small intestine may be expedited by giving a subcutaneous injection of prostigmine (Friedenberg *et al.*, 1962). The small intestinal study is carried out (*a*) when a barium enema has failed to reflux into the terminal ileum; (*b*) to determine the extent of the disease within the small intestine; and more specifically (*c*) in order to find out if skip lesions are present. Unfortunately some of the earliest changes noticed in the ileum, such as hypermotility and spasm, are entirely non-specific. Again screening is more important than spot films. Non-filling of part of the intestine may be of no significance. However, its *persistence* at a second examination some weeks later is strongly suggestive of a skip lesion.

(4) *Fistulography*
Gastrografin (endografin) is the safest contrast medium to use for demonstrating a fistulous tract. A thin barium suspension can be run in through a balloon catheter when it is judged that there is no risk of its entering soft tissues or a serosal cavity. In Crohn's disease, a fistula is mostly long, indirect and with narrowed segments along its course. As a result the success rate of fistulography is not very high. Many fistulae are in the region of the pelvis and perineum, so that the gonads of a young patient are likely to be irradiated.

(5) *Angiography*
Selective mesenteric arteriography can demonstrate the vascular architecture in the intestine. At the present time in inflammatory bowel disease the technique is in the development stage. It is being used for special research purposes but not as a routine diagnostic aid. It may be of value in the differential diagnosis between Crohn's disease and vascular lesions of the bowel.

(6) *Other Radiological Investigations*
Intravenous pyelography is useful in the small number of patients with Crohn's disease who have obstructive uropathy or renal calculi. Cholecystography is indicated when gall-stones are suspected either at the time of detecting the bowel inflammation or years after intestinal resection (page 134). Occasionally ascending lymphangiography is desirable when a reticulosis has to be excluded.

Radiological Changes
(1) Small Intestine
The earliest change in the small intestine is some blunting and distortion of the valvulae, which may be shown up when barium refluxes into the terminal ileum. The appearance may be asymmetrical and is probably accounted for by oedema in the deeper parts of the intestinal wall.

Like many of the radiological changes in Crohn's disease, by itself it cannot be regarded as specific. Any inflammatory lesion or lymphatic obstruction might give a similar appearance. There is some rigidity of the affected part of the wall. This is easier to assess on screening. It becomes increasingly significant when it is detected on repeated films

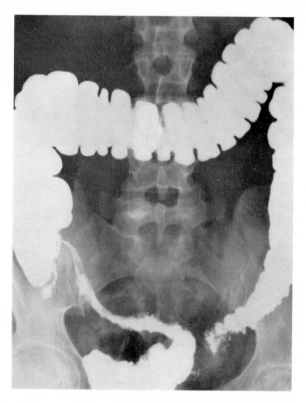

Fig. 1. Barium enema showing Crohn's disease of the distal ileum, with contact involvement of the sigmoid loop. There is irregular narrowing of the ileum which is rigid and arranged as a wide arc.

and on films taken obliquely. Sometimes there is rather persistent irregularity of the lumen without distortion of the valvulae (Marshak and Linder, 1970). There may be little interference with peristalsis. Spasm and hypermotility can make it difficult to outline the lower ileum; they are more troublesome in children and can give a misleading impression. If there is any doubt, a repeat examination should be performed 2 or 3 weeks later. Persistence of any irregularity or other abnormality is very strong evidence in favour of organic disease.

These above-mentioned changes are early; many patients will already have progressed to a more chronic stage in their disease when they are first examined radiologically. By this time 6–8 cm of lower ileum may be clearly involved (Fig. 1). Ulceration may now be visible. When the

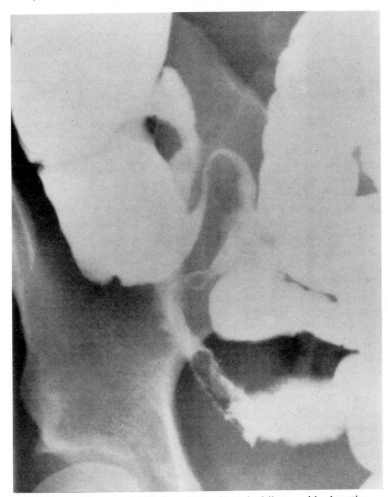

FIG. 2. Rigid, reversed "S" disposition of terminal ileum, with ulceration and spiculation (bottom). The appendix is filled.

disease has been present for a long time ulceration is discernible in 80 per cent of cases (Fig. 2). With the inflammatory cell infiltrate in the wall, rigidity will be more marked, and will no longer be confused with spasm. The luminal outline becomes irregular; in nearly two-thirds of all cases the irregularities of outline are finally 1–2 mm deep. Characteristically the terminal ileum frequently resembles a reversed and elongated letter "S". Very fine clefts or fissures at right angles to the lumen are occasionally seen ("spiculation"). Most radiologists would say that they are less common and less easy to identify than in the colon, but when present they are very suggestive of Crohn's disease.

Between the longitudinal streaks and transverse clefts of the ulcerated mucosa somewhat oedematous islands of epithelial tissue may survive, and on barium examination they sometimes present a cobblestone appearance. This is not easy to demonstrate and is said to be best seen in the jejunum (Marshak and Linder, 1970). It relies on a subjective impression and is not a particularly reliable sign. As ulceration proceeds, the whole wall becomes denuded, and with concomitant fibrosis, the lumen is progressively narrowed. Eventually the stenosis causes increasing obstruction to the onward passage of luminal contents. The intestine proximal to the main lesion becomes dilated (2·5 cm or more in diameter) or in the jejunum pulsion diverticula may form (Fig. 3). The abnormality in the wall of the small intestine may extend a long distance proximal to the upper limit of ulceration. There is likely to be malabsorption in patients with this type of very widespread jejuno-ileal involvement. Malabsorption causes stippling or clumping of barium and loss of the uniform, feathery appearance of the contrast medium which is seen in the upper and middle portions of the small intestine in healthy subjects.

Although in 80 per cent of cases Crohn's disease mainly affects the small intestine, nevertheless there is often noticeable deformity of the adjacent caecum when it is studied radiologically. The lower pole of the caecum looks as if it were gripped and squeezed by some unseen hand. The ascending colon beyond is sometimes indented from one side. Distortion or loss of distensibility of the caecum was observed in about 1 in 3 of the Aberdeen patients. In spite of the probable involvement of the caecal wall by the granulomatous process, it is not at all unusual to obtain good filling of the appendix.

Skip lesions, well away from the main granulomatous mass, are only present in approximately 10 per cent of patients. When present they are often multiple, but each lesion is usually short. They are therefore difficult to delineate on barium follow through studies. Attention tends to be centred on the distal ileum, and a short skip lesion in jejunum may easily be missed unless it is causing marked stenosis or the related mucosa is oedematous. Between adjacent skip lesions the intervening, pliable, small intestine may appear suspended, like a hammock.

Fistulae rarely show up on barium studies. Most fistulae in Crohn's disease are narrow, tortuous, and only open intermittently. There is little chance of barium being able to outline the full extent of a fistula, although the point of origin from the intestine is sometimes revealed.

External fistulae are better outlined by fistulography, particularly when a fine Foley bag catheter can be inserted in the orifice. A wide, direct internal fistula must not be confused with an earlier surgical short-circuiting procedure. Old operation notes may not be clear as to which parts were anastomosed. Indeed within the abdomen of some patients

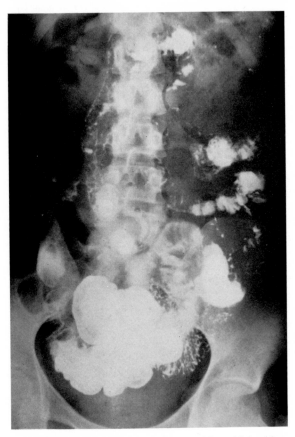

FIG. 3. Pseudo-diverticulae in Crohn's disease with multiple skip areas in the jejunum (left upper abdomen).

who have had numerous operations for advanced Crohn's disease, it may be very difficult for the surgeon to tell precisely what parts of the intestine he is joining together.

Kantor's Sign. It was the appearance of the rigid, narrowed terminal ileum, with its surface irregularity, which led Kantor (1934) to describe it as resembling a piece of frayed cotton string. Although somewhat unpopular in post-war years, this is still an apt description of advanced Crohn's disease. In 1970, Dyer and his colleagues reported the results of an evaluation of the incidence and reliability of radiographic signs in the small intestinal type of Crohn's disease. Two separate radiologists, who were unaware of the details of the patients, wrote down their assessment of the common radiological features seen on the follow through films from 50 patients with ileal disease. Visualization of the terminal ileum was good in 70–80 per cent of cases. The conclusions arrived at after comparing the radiologists' reports were that rigidity and contraction of the bowel wall, with surface irregularity and ulceration, were the most consistent and valuable signs of Crohn's disease. When present, clefts (spicules) provided strong confirmatory evidence. Rigidity, noted on at least 3 films, was present in only 26 per cent of the series studied by Dyer *et al.* (1970) whereas they detected spiculation in 60 per cent of the films of diseased ileum. The cobblestone mucosal appearance and stenosis were present in more than 25 per cent of cases, but were subject to considerable observer variation. Infrequent signs, with wide disagreement between radiologists, included slight irregularities and a featureless appearance of the mucosa, longitudinal streaking of the wall, and the presence (or otherwise) of skip areas and fistulae. Although not often demonstrated, the last two features scarcely ever occur in any other disease of the small intestine.

Other Findings. The considerable thickening of the mesentery and marked lymphadenopathy that are so often observed in Crohn's disease cause the loops of the lower small intestine to become separate from one another. Instead of being arranged in their normal serpentine disposition, they are seen to lie in rather fixed arcs some distance apart, like rigid festoons (Fig. 4). A large abscess in the right lower abdomen is unusual in Crohn's disease. If one does develop, a rather oedematous loop of intestine may be stretched over it in a fixed and unchanging position. It is much more common to find one or more loops of ileum adherent to the apex of the sigmoid part of the colon, which itself may show clear radiological evidence of Crohn's disease.

Recurrent Disease

Even the most skilful surgeon would have very great difficulty in joining the ends of bowel together so neatly that radiologically the area looked completely normal. Many of the irregularities seen in the vicinity of any anastomosis are man-made, not the result of disease. Great caution must therefore be exercised in interpreting post-operative barium examinations.

It is not uncommon to find that between 2 and 5 years after an anastomosis has been fashioned, cicatricial contracture slowly narrows the opening, causing some obstruction and the return of colicky abdominal pain. If the obstruction is of mechanical type only, the ileum immediately proximal to the narrowed ring should be distensible and moderately dilated on barium enema (or small bowel follow through) examination. When narrowing at a stoma is due to recurrent Crohn's disease, the

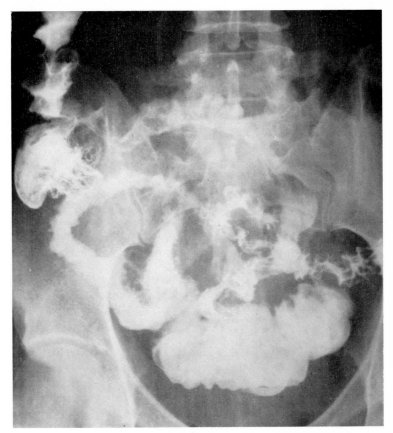

FIG. 4. Separation of festoon-like loops of lower ileum resulting from thickening of the mesentery, and lymphadenopathy.

adjacent ileum is likely to be narrowed, rigid and irregular, as in primary small intestinal disease. Recurrence is more common and more obvious proximal to an anastomosis, but in some patients it does develop on the distal side. The patient's general condition may remain good, and belie the radiological appearances.

One set of circumstances can mimic the radiological evidence of recurrent disease. When a primary resection and anastomosis has been followed by local sepsis and fistula formation, there is likely to be permanent distortion and narrowing of the joined portions of intestine. Fibrosis and dense adhesions firmly tether them to the rigid posterior wall of the iliac fossa. When scarring alone is responsible for the narrowing, the ESR should be normal and the stool occult blood test negative. If recurrent Crohn's disease has developed, selective angiography (page 104) may reveal hypervascularity in the affected region.

Colonic Disease

The clinical picture of Crohn's disease of the colon has been recognized for little more than a decade. During this comparatively short period the radiological features have been closely studied and evaluated. The radiological appearances are now well defined (Lockhart-Mummery and Morson, 1964; Capek *et al.*, 1968; Fry and Stanley, 1971). The pathological process would seem to be essentially similar to that in the ileum, modified only by the much greater circumference and relatively less muscular wall of the colon. Submucosal oedema is followed by ulceration, transmural inflammatory cell infiltration and fissure formation (spiculation). This resumé of the pathology of the condition may be an over-simplification. The term "Crohn's disease of the colon" may embrace several related but slightly different conditions. At the present time we do not know how to distinguish between them.

The most helpful signs on barium enema examination are the following—

   (i) Right-sided disease, with sparing of the rectum. The other common ulcerative disease of the colon, idiopathic ulcerative proctocolitis, mostly appears first and is most severe in the distal colon and rectum.

   (ii) Discontinuity, with skip lesions. Short ulcerated and narrowed segments are usually separated from each other by many centimetres of normal colon.

   (iii) Ileal involvement (Fig. 5). If a characteristic narrow, rigid and irregular lesion is shown in the terminal ileum, then any abnormality demonstrated in the colon is very likely to be Crohn's disease.

   (iv) Asymmetry of lesion (Fig. 6). In the earlier stages only part of the circumference may be diseased, the remaining part retaining its normal appearance and distensibility. At operation the early lesion may resemble a greatly thickened taenia several centimetres long.

   (v) Spiculation. Rose-thorn fissures extending deep into the colon wall are characteristic (Fig. 7). In the past they may have been misinterpreted as the "saw-tooth" appearance of pre-diverticulosis. Because many of the patients are over the age of 50 years, co-existent diverticula are quite common.

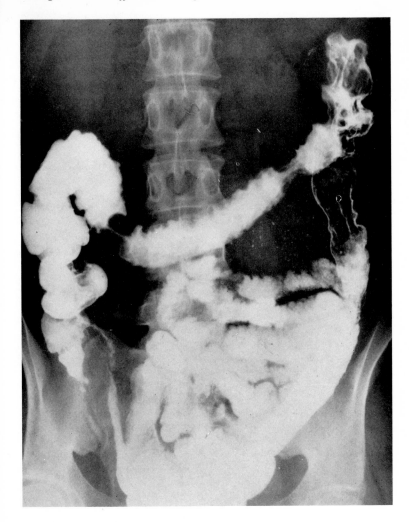

FIG. 5. Crohn's disease of the terminal ileum and transverse colon. The lesions are discontinuous. There are stenoses at both ends of the sausage-shaped colonic segment.

(vi) Fistula formation. Apart from advanced carcinoma and diverticulitis, very few colonic diseases give rise to fistulae into the bladder, vagina or to the abdominal wall or perianal region. The fistula is the eventual outcome of a rose-thorn fissure which has penetrated right through the wall of the colon.

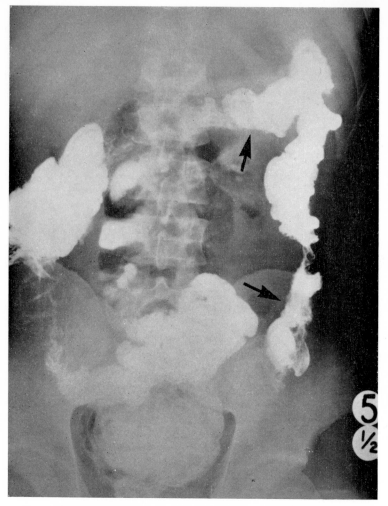

FIG. 6. Asymmetrical involvement of the colon by Crohn's disease. At laparotomy there were granulomatous plaques on the central aspect of the descending and transverse colon (arrows).

The other changes in colonic Crohn's disease are less specific and consequently less helpful. With oedema in the submucosa the contrast medium in the lumen may look as though it has been indented from various directions by a series of thumb-prints. The combination of mucosal oedema with fine linear ulcers and transverse fissures some-times gives the reticulated, cobblestone appearance (Fig. 8) described in the ileum. Minor mucosal abnormalities are usually best seen on post-evacuation films. Considerable disorganization of the mucosal folds may be noted. A variety of inflammatory and vascular diseases can produce similar changes.

Ulceration can be extensive. There is a tendency for the ulcers to run in the long axis of the colon, with connecting transverse fissures. On

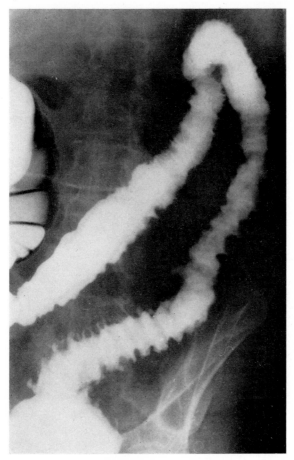

FIG. 7. Spiculation (rose-thorn fissures) in Crohn's disease of the sigmoid, descending and transverse colon. There is thumb-printing on the lateral aspect of the descending colon.

opening a resected specimen, the pattern resembles that of a railway track. Ulcers may be up to 3 mm deep. Collar-stud abscesses (Fig. 9) are by no means uncommon; they are certainly not pathognomonic of proctocolitis. In a few patients with colonic Crohn's disease a double-contour effect may be produced.

With the much greater diameter of the colon compared to the ileum and more undermining, surviving islets of mucosa in an ulcerated area sometimes assume the form of pseudo-polyps. However, the latter are more common in proctocolitis. When there is a temporary remission

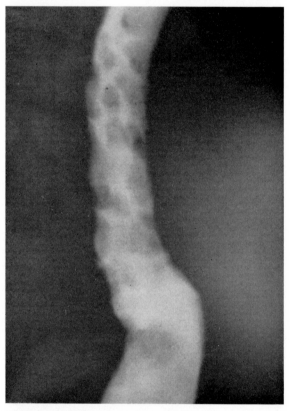

FIG. 8. Cobblestone appearance in the descending colon. It is not diagnostic of Crohn's disease.

and fibrosis takes place, a strictured segment appears. In the absence of any skip lesions, it can be very difficult at a single examination to differentiate such a stricture from one caused by a stenosing carcinoma or by healing ischaemic colitis.

When there is considerable thickening of the wall of the transverse colon there may be a noticeable space between the barium in the lumen and air that is present in the patient's stomach (Cummack, 1969). It is well known that in ulcerative colitis the retro-rectal space is frequently increased. One in three patients with Crohn's disease in the distal large bowel also shows an increase in the space between rectum and sacrum, but the change is less pronounced than in proctocolitis (Eklöf and Gierup, 1970).

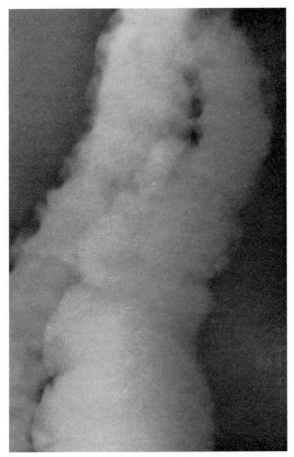

Fig. 9. Collar-stud abscesses in Crohn's disease at the splenic flexure. They can give a double-contour effect.

Modern techniques now enable an experienced radiologist to make a correct diagnosis of Crohn's disease of the colon in between 80 and 90 per cent of cases. One of the interesting observations is the speed at which change within the colon can take place (Jones *et al.*, 1969; Brahme and Wenckert, 1970). Sequential examinations in some of the Aberdeen patients have shown diseased areas extending and new skip lesions appearing within a matter of weeks. Under effective medical therapy regression has been equally rapid and dramatic.

Selective Mesenteric Angiography

In Crohn's disease, mesenteric angiography is mainly used in research. It may be of value in the clinical situation (*a*) to exclude vascular lesions of the intestine; (*b*) in elucidating the cause of persistent anaemia; (*c*) in suspected recurrent disease, when barium studies are equivocal and there are strong reasons for not re-exploring the abdomen.

Earlier work suggested that with active Crohn's disease in ileum or colon there was hypervascularity while in the late, fibrotic stages the blood supply to the wall was diminished (Lunderquist *et al.*, 1967). The hypervascularity (Potocky *et al.*, 1968; Brahme and Wenckert, 1970) was demonstrated by the leash of small arteries supplying the affected segment, with increased flow, by the dense blush in the intestinal wall during the capillary phase, and by rapid filling of the veins (normally they may not be visualized). In the arterial phase the terminal branches of the superior mesenteric artery are kinked and spread apart, probably by the thickening and oedema in the mesentery. When there is foreshortening of the wall by long-standing fibrosis the terminal branches arising from the juxta-mural arcade look bunched together. Because of the increased thickness of the wall the vasa rectae are wider, longer and more tortuous. By injection studies of excised specimens and micro-angiography Brahme (1971) has shown that, in severe disease, there are numerous vessels in the submucosa and in the subserosa, with tortuous vascular channels between the two layers. Vascular supply was most abundant close to ulcers, fissures and areas of cobblestone formation. The more severe the disease the greater was the degree of hypervascularity.

Brahme's *in vivo* studies had sometimes shown hypovascularity in the terminal ileum. However, examination of injected specimens revealed many patent vessels, with very little evidence of thrombosis or vas-culitis. Possible explanations of the seemingly poor perfusion of the terminal ileum are that: (1) the pressure gradient along the length of the superior mesenteric artery prevents an adequate amount of blood from reaching the large vascular bed in the distal ileum; (2) oedema in the mesentery increases the peripheral resistance distally; and (3) that with inflammation in the mesentery itself there may be rapid transfer of blood from the arterial to the venous side before it reaches the ileal wall ("mesenteric steal").

Nutritional Disturbances

The nutritional disturbances from which a proportion of patients with Crohn's disease suffer frequently are not the result of malabsorption alone. In most cases they have a multifactorial origin. Inadequate food intake must always be considered first. Faulty dietary habits are some-times to blame, especially among older people living alone. Not only is the calorie content insufficient but their food lacks essential substances such as iron and vitamins. Fear of precipitating a bout of intestinal colic stops some patients from eating as much as they otherwise would. Nausea and vomiting, which appear when a degree of intestinal obstruction develops, inevitably lead to malnutrition.

Fluid and electrolytes may be lost in the vomitus. There can be large losses of sodium in the severe diarrhoea of ulcerative proctocolitis. Fortunately in Crohn's disease diarrhoea mostly is not excessive in its daily frequency. It has often been present for many months or years, so that gradually body stores of sodium and potassium have become depleted. Serious losses of blood and albumin can take place from the ulcerated wall of diseased small intestine. Some authors cite external fistulae as being an important factor in the losses sustained by a few patients with Crohn's disease. Today they should be uncommon, and a fistula that is constantly pouring out large quantities of intestinal contents is almost always due to some surgical error or misadventure. A spontaneous internal fistula can cause excessively rapid passage of food through the gastrointestinal tract.

Malabsorption itself depends on and varies with the following factors—

(1) The severity of the mucosal damage and whether any absorptive power remains.
(2) The site of the lesion. Carbohydrates and folate for example are normally absorbed in the jejunum, and vitamin B_{12} and bile salts in the distal ileum.
(3) The extent of the disease in the small intestine. Crohn's disease in the colon causes little interference with absorption, apart from water and sodium (Head *et al.*, 1969). Diffuse jejuno-ileal disease causes very severe malabsorption.
(4) Transit time, which may be increased.
(5) Surgical procedures. Resections, particularly if repeated, may significantly reduce the absorptive area available. Entero-anastomoses often cause blind loops, which (rarely) may cause malabsorption from bacterial proliferation.
(6) Loss of co-factors, such as bile salts, that are necessary for the absorption of fat.
(7) Deficient secretion from accessory glands. In unoperated cases gastric acid output usually is normal (Fielding *et al.*, 1971), but in chronic cases of Crohn's disease it is possible that there are defects in hepatic and pancreatic secretion. Further studies are necessary.

Even when there is adequate food intake and reasonable absorptive capacity, increased catabolism resulting from inflammation in the intestine and possibly adjacent sepsis may then result in slow deterioration in nutritional status.

The results quoted in the following paragraphs are based partly on the reports in the literature and partly on the Aberdeen experience. Other workers have not always distinguished between patients who have had and those who have not had a definitive operation, and frequently the site of the disease has not been defined. A hospital doctor—and particularly a surgeon—does not often see a new case of Crohn's disease that has not already received some treatment from a family doctor. If antibiotics or corticosteroids have been given they may markedly alter the picture of malabsorption.

Weight. At the time of diagnosis nearly 30 per cent of the Aberdeen patients stated that they were within 3 kg of what they regarded as their normal weight. Regular weighing is valuable in the assessment and management of Crohn's disease. An unintentional weight loss of up to 10 kg in a 12-month period is not uncommon. A loss in excess of 15 kg was reported by 14 per cent of the patients and must be regarded as serious. Detailed study of the patient's intake and absorptive capacity are indicated and energetic replacement therapy is necessary.

Haemoglobin. Some degree of iron-deficiency anaemia is almost universal in patients who have had symptoms for more than one month. When the small bowel was involved, in 83 patients in Aberdeen the mean haemoglobin value was 10·4 gm per 100 ml when first seen (range 8·6–14·3 gm). In 30 patients with colonic disease mean Hb value was lower, 10·1 gm (range 7·3–14 gm). None of these patients had had a major haemorrhage. The degree of activity of the disease in these patients is not known for certain, but as the estimations were made at their first hospital attendance, presumably the bowel disease was in an active stage in the majority. Fielding (1971) noted that 24 out of 36 patients with active Crohn's disease had a Hb of less than 12·5 gm per 100 ml; during the quiescent phase only 1 patient in 6 was below this level. The Hb changes were reflected in the serum iron levels. Nearly 66 per cent of those with active disease had less than 50 micrograms per 100 ml, compared to only 24 per cent with such low levels during quiescent periods. Tygat *et al.* (1967) also noticed low serum iron levels during exacerbations. As iron is absorbed mainly in the duodenum and upper jejunum, rare sites for Crohn's disease, the iron-deficiency anaemia in most instances is caused by persistent loss of small quantities of blood in the faeces.

Serum Folate. An adequate intake is necessary to maintain a normal level in serum or whole blood. In 12 untreated Aberdeen patients with localized ileal disease, the serum folate, estimated by microbiological assay using *Lactobacillus casei*, fell below the normal range of 6–20 micrograms/ml in 10 cases. This is in agreement with the findings of

Hoffbrand *et al.* (1968). Studying 64 patients (40 had been operated on), they found subnormal serum folates in 81 per cent; 42 per cent of their control subjects also had subnormal levels. Seven out of 19 patients in the St Bartholomew's Hospital series had low concentrations of red cell folate, varying with the severity of the disease. Smith (1971) also found serum folate levels frequently to be abnormally low. However, Dotevall and Kock (1968) reported normal serum levels in 38 per cent and normal whole blood folate levels in 72 per cent of their patients.

Vitamin B_{12} Absorption. The Schilling test is most often performed by estimating the percentage of the labelled dose of B_{12} that is excreted in the urine in 24 hours, the usual lower limit being 7·5 per cent. Some workers take a different limit, and many include a broad band of borderline values, making any comparison difficult. Whole-body counting would be more accurate. Resection of about 90 cm of terminal ileum can profoundly affect B_{12} absorption (Fone *et al.*, 1961; Schofield, 1967); few surgeons today would be foolish enough to attempt to achieve a cure by removing longer lengths of small intestine. Dotevall and Kock (1968) in Goteborg had only 4 abnormal results in 19 patients. In Aberdeen 3 out of 12 patients with ileal disease had defective absorption, but in Edinburgh 9 out of 12 patients with Crohn's disease of ileum had abnormal Schilling tests (Smith, 1971). There is some evidence that the results of the Schilling test of B_{12} absorption may improve some months after bypass surgery (Nygaard *et al.*, 1970).

Serum B_{12} Concentrations. The concentrations nearly always fall within the normal range of 100–720 pg/ml unless long lengths of ileum have been removed (Schofield, 1967; Hoffbrand *et al.*, 1968). Twenty-one out of 23 Aberdeen patients with Crohn's disease of the small intestine had normal values prior to operation, and all 7 colonic patients examined also had normal serum concentrations.

Only 5–7 per cent of patients, including those who have had resections, go on to develop megaloblastic anaemia after 5 years (Steinberg, 1961). Untreated and following extensive resection, it is possible for a patient to develop sub-acute combined degeneration of the spinal cord (Best, 1959).

White Blood Cell Changes. In most patients the WBC count is within the range 5,000–12,000 cu mm. Sepsis, fistulae and abscesses increase the count. A slight eosinophilia up to 10 per cent has been reported (Smith, 1967) but it is rather inconstant. During an active stage of the disease there is hypersegmentation of the polymorphs (Hoffbrand, *et al.*, 1968). In a few patients there may be abnormal circulating lymphocytes, amounting to almost one-third of the total count (Smith, 1967), and a relative monocytosis. Thrombocytosis has also been described (Moro-witz *et al.*, 1968). Apart from the effects produced by bacterial infection, the differential count of the white blood cells has not shown any unusual variations in the Aberdeen series of patients.

Plasma Proteins. There is considerable loss of protein from the ulcerated gut, the severity of the loss depending on the extent and activity of the disease (Beeken, 1969). Hypoproteinaemia results, being reflected mainly in a reduction in the serum albumin concentration (Steinfeld *et al.*, 1960). The mean value for serum albumin in 54 Aberdeen patients with Crohn's disease in varying sites before treatment was 3·3 gm/100 ml (range 2·1–4·5 gm). This value is considerably higher than the 2·1 gm/100 ml quoted by Smith (1971), but as his patients were extensively investigated they may have had unusually severe disease. There is good correlation between disease activity and low serum albumin levels (Fielding, 1971). An abnormally high proportion of the body albumin lies in the intravascular compartment in Crohn's disease (Bendixen *et al.*, 1968). Removal of the site of protein loss effects considerable improvement.

The reduction in serum albumin may be matched by a slight increase in the globulin fraction (Hansing and Meeuwisse, 1971). The A:G ratio in the Aberdeen patients was 1:1, but in active disease it is frequently reversed. The immunoglobulins have been considered on page 39. The relationship between variations in the immunoglobulin fractions and the duration, extent and severity of Crohn's disease has still to be determined and their significance established. According to Weeke and Jarnum (1971) the ocosomucoid and haptoglobulin fractions are increased in active Crohn's disease; they observed a pronounced elevation of haptoglobulin when fistulae and abscesses were present.

Erythrocyte Sedimentation Rate. The ESR is a non-specific but easily performed estimate of the degree of activity of various pathological processes that may affect the rate of sedimentation of the red blood cells. Readings at the time of admission to hospital were available for 104 out of the 175 Aberdeen patients. The ESR was not always measured in the earlier years of the study or in those patients who had emergency operations. The reading was below 20 mm/hour in 19 cases. The mean value in the remaining 85 patients was 48 mm/hour (range 20–104 mm); in almost two-thirds of these patients the ESR was between 30 mm and 65 mm/hour; later in the course of their disease higher readings were sometimes recorded. In Uppsala 85 per cent of the patients studied by Krause *et al.* (1971) had an ESR in excess of 20 mm/hour.

While a normal ESR certainly does not exclude the possibility of Crohn's disease, raised values probably are an imprecise guide to activity and to the effects of therapy. The author believes that it is unwise to undertake elective surgery until medical treatment has reduced the ESR significantly and preferably below 50 mm/hour. Unfortunately there would not appear to be any correlation between the initial ESR and the later development of recurrent disease (see Chap. X).

Other Biochemical Parameters. The Birmingham workers attach considerable importance to the serum seromucoids (Cooke *et al.*, 1958). In 27 out of 35 patients with active Crohn's disease the concentration exceeded 150 mg/100 ml; only 10 out of 133 patients whose disease was inactive showed such high values, the difference between the two groups being highly significant. This biochemical estimation is only undertaken by a few laboratories.

Low serum sodium levels will be detected in patients with prolonged or copious diarrhoea (Atwell, 1964). Approximately half of the patients with extensive active disease show hypokalaemia; there may be other reasons for their lassitude and flaccid, distended appearance. In nearly all patients serum calcium is normal (Harris *et al.*, 1970); some years ago it had been stated that one-quarter of all patients had hypocalcaemia (Jackson, 1958). It is very rare indeed for symptoms of tetany to occur in uncomplicated disease. About 5 per cent have low magnesium concentrations, less than 1·5 mEq/L (Gerlach, 1970). Serum concentrations are not a very good index of the biochemical status of the patient. The symptoms and signs of hypomagnesaemia are confused by those of other co-existent deficiencies; they include confusion, agitation and athetoid movements. Magnesium and calcium losses are in proportion to the degree of steatorrhoea present (Booth *et al.*, 1963).

When the liver becomes damaged in chronic Crohn's disease, there will be derangement of the liver function tests (page 131). Hypocholesterolaemia was present in more than half of the patients investigated by Dyer and Dawson (1971). It was independent of site, steatorrhoea or resection, but did appear to be related to disease activity.

Steatorrhoea. A recently passed stool should be inspected in the bedpan; its colour and consistence are noted and also the presence of any blood, pus or mucus. When a patient has steatorrhoea the stool is pale, bulky and tends to float on water. It has an offensive odour. With the intestinal irritation and hurry resulting from Crohn's disease, the stool is frequently unformed even though it contains an excessive amount of unabsorbed fat.

Careful in-patient balance studies are necessary in order to make an accurate estimate of faecal fat losses. A standard 100 gm fat diet is given, and after a 2-day equilibration period (or check on transit by oral carmine marker) the collection of faeces is carried out for a 3-day or 5-day period. Failure to re-absorb bile salts from diseased lower ileum almost certainly contributes to the patient's inability to absorb fat properly (Badley *et al.*, 1969). Pancreatic deficiency may play some part, but the principal defect is in the unhealthy intestinal mucosa, especially in the jejunum.

Ninety per cent of patients with extensive jejuno-ileal disease lose more than 5 gm of fat per 24 hours in the faeces (Smith, 1971). Three Aberdeen patients who at laparotomy were shown to have disease throughout most of the small intestine had a mean loss of 8·1 gm per 24 hours. With ileal disease alone such losses are uncommon; only 6 out of 19 exceeded the normal faecal output. Twelve of the 21 patients with Crohn's disease studied by Cooke (1955) had steatorrhoea. He considered that it indicated widespread mucosal abnormality and heralded a poor prognosis.

Pimparkar *et al.* (1960) stated that steatorrhoea was common in Crohn's disease, but the site and number of complications and operations were not clearly defined. Only 40 per cent of the Goteborg patients had normal fat excretion (Dotevall and Kock, 1968); another 28 per cent were regarded as borderline rather than having frank steatorrhoea. Twelve of the 30 patients in this Swedish series had had operations.

Half of the Edinburgh patients with widespread disease and steatorrhoea were also losing more than 2 gm of nitrogen per day in their faeces (Smith, 1971) from the breakdown of protein.

Faecal Occult Blood. With ulcerative, exudative disease in the intestine, small amounts of blood are regularly being shed into the intestinal lumen. Three tests for occult blood in the faeces should be carried out over a period of days. One or two may be negative. However, it is rare when the ileum is diseased to get 3 negative results. With colonic involvement the test is much more likely to be positive.

Other Absorption Tests. Chalfin and Holt (1968) obtained evidence of lactase deficiency on oral lactose tests in 3 out of 5 patients with Crohn's disease. Such frequent lactose malabsorption was not confirmed by Gudmand-Hoyer and Jarnum (1970) who found only a 6 per cent incidence in 71 patients. The latter workers did observe that 3 out of 9 patients benefited from a milk-free diet even though they had not had lactose malabsorption.

The d-xylose absorption test is nearly always normal in Crohn's disease unless almost the entire jejunum and ileum are damaged by the granulomatous process (Chanarin and Bennett, 1962; Dotevall and Kock, 1968).

Sigmoidoscopy and Rectal Biopsy
Any patient suspected of having Crohn's disease or any other inflammatory condition of the intestinal tract should have a sigmoidoscopy. It is the author's practice to complete the examination by taking a

biopsy specimen of rectal mucosa and submucosa, using crocodile biopsy forceps.

There should be no special preparation of the bowel before making the first attempt to pass the sigmoidoscope. Suppositories and enemas only alter the mucosal appearance and render interpretation more difficult. As most patients with Crohn's disease have diarrhoea, the rectum and lower sigmoid are generally empty. It is unusual for the bowel to be so loaded with faeces that a preliminary washout is necessary in order to obtain a clear view.

Before passing the instrument the perianal region is inspected and a digital rectal examination performed. There may be discoloration of the skin, and the orifice of a fistula, or the scar of a long-forgotten ischiorectal abscess may be seen. Digital examination helps to exclude a rectal carcinoma or polyp, and provides a faecal smear that can be tested for occult blood.

The rigid metal sigmoidoscope usually passes easily in patients with Crohn's disease confined to the small intestine. When the frequency of bowel movements is no greater than 3 or 4 times per day, there is little trouble from liquid faeces flooding down from above—this can be a problem in ulcerative proctocolitis. The mucosa of the rectum and lower sigmoid, up to 25 cm, looks intact and is a uniform pale pink colour. Some excess mucus is sometimes noticed on the surface. The rectal walls distend away readily on air insufflation. In patients with more frequent diarrhoea the lower 2–4 cm of the rectum frequently look decidedly red, hyperaemic, and irritated, while the upper rectum is normal. If the lower part of the rectum is fiery red in colour, with a friable mucosa and some muco-pus on its surface, then this appearance probably represents the start of Crohn's disease in that patient's rectum.

The rectum and lower sigmoid are involved in almost one-half of all patients with Crohn's disease in the colon. The mucosa is inflamed and oedematous and may show a cobblestone surface or discrete ulcers. Mucopus is obvious but fresh blood is less often seen. The walls become rigid and indistensible and the lumen is distorted. Many of these patients with distal colonic disease will have fissures and fistulae around the anus, so that manipulation of the instrument can be very painful. In such cases, if a good view has not been obtained, it may be wiser to give the patient a short general anaesthetic before another sigmoidoscopy is attempted. The bladder can be emptied and a bimanual examination of the pelvis be carried out under the anaesthetic.

Physicians seem rather loth to wield the biting biopsy forceps used by surgeons (Morson, 1971). They prefer suction biopsies. A modified and rigid version of Wood's originally flexible gastric biopsy tube is generally employed (Dick *et al.*, 1970). A negative pressure of 10–20 cm Hg is applied before the blade slices off the portion of mucosa that has been

drawn into the eyes of the tube, together with a small circle of underlying submucosa. Three or four biopsies are taken from different parts
of the rectum. The submucosal surface of each biopsy specimen is then
gently applied and pressed on to the frosted surface of a special glass
slide. The slide is placed in a fixative such as saturated solution of
mercuric chloride in 10 per cent formalin or in formalin alone. This
technique is said to give better orientation of the specimen for the
pathologist.

After having a rectal biopsy performed, the patient is warned that he
may notice slight rectal bleeding during the next 24 hours. No barium
enema examination should be carried out for at least 48 hours after
taking a rectal or sigmoid biopsy.

Histological Findings on Rectal Biopsy. The most significant findings
(Morson, 1971) in a small rectal biopsy in Crohn's disease are, in order
of importance—

(1) Disproportionate submucosal infiltration by chronic inflammatory cells compared to the relatively intact mucosa.
(2) Epithelioid cell granulomas, with or without giant cells.
(3) Fissure formation, into the submucosa or deeper layers.

There is no doubt that abnormal tissue can be obtained from a
rectum which looks normal through the sigmoidoscope (Present *et al.*,
1967). Numerous examples of this seeming discrepancy have been
observed in Aberdeen patients. The less normal the surface appears, the
greater will be the chance of finding significant changes in the submucosa. Anderson and Bogoch (1968) noted that with small bowel
disease, what they termed non-specific changes were present in 43 per
cent of rectal biopsy specimens. In a study of 79 patients, Dyer *et al.*
(1970) confirmed this percentage, noted the lack of correlation with the
colour and texture of the surface, but felt that the infiltration with
lymphocytes, plasma cells and eosinophils indicated the presence of
organic disease in the more proximal part of the intestine. When a
perianal lesion, such as a fistula, was present in ileal Crohn's disease,
the rectal biopsy findings were always diagnostic, with marked submucosal infiltration, granulomas, fissures, etc.

Abnormal biopsies are obtained from nearly 75 per cent of patients
with Crohn's disease in the colon. In less than half of these abnormal
specimens the findings are again characteristic of Crohn's disease; in the
remainder there are non-specific changes such as surface ulceration,
hyperaemia, submucosal inflammation or crypt abscesses. The closer
the lesion in the large bowel is to the anal canal, the higher becomes the
proportion of diagnostic changes. With ano-rectal Crohn's disease
virtually every biopsy specimen will show the changes that Morson
regards as being most significant.

Quite apart from the pathological changes that they may reveal, intestinal biopsy specimens may be used for studies on enzymes and other substances. Histochemical methods have been developed for visualizing and measuring neutral mucins and mucosubstances. There is a marked decrease in the mucosubstance content of the mucosa in patients with active ulcerative protocolitis; no such decrease occurs in Crohn's disease (Filipe and Dawson, 1970).

Colonoscopy. There is little difficulty in passing the flexible Olympus CF fiberoptic colonoscope for a distance of 35–40 cm in to the colon (Dean and Shearman, 1970; Kyle, 1971). One or two preparatory bowel washouts with 2–3 litres of water are needed in patients who do not have diarrhoea. Sedation and analgesia are obtained by administering pethidine or diazepan and propanthine (up to 30 mg intramuscularly) may be injected to counteract spasm in the colon. The advancing tip of the colonoscope is usually halted at the apex of the sigmoid loop or junction of descending and sigmoid colon. Beyond 40 cm in a diseased bowel it can be difficult to flex the tip or advance it by pushing from behind, particularly when the lumen is narrowed by chronic inflammation. Occasionally the instrument will pass smoothly up to the splenic flexure. Judged by 2 years' experience of its use, the colonoscope would appear to be of value in the diagnosis of polyps and other small tumours of the colon. The specimen obtained with the biopsy forceps is tiny. It may be sufficient for histological purposes when the specimen is taken from a projecting lesion, but is less satisfactory when taken from a flat surface. Colonoscopy may be of limited value in inflammatory disease of the left colon. Salmon *et al.* (1971) are rather more optimistic about its use, while Nagasako and his Japanese colleagues (1971) claim to have been able to biopsy the terminal ileum in 30 patients through the colonoscope.

Peroral Intestinal Biopsy. With a Crosby type capsule it is possible to obtain confirmation of the diagnosis of Crohn's disease from the upper small intestine (Harrer *et al.*, 1970; Hermos *et al.*, 1970). Laparotomy may thereby be avoided or at least postponed for a time while medical therapy is given a fair trial. Biopsy specimens from jejunum are often normal when the disease is in the ileum. However, specimens with typical granulomas are sometimes obtained from jejunum which radiologically looks perfectly normal (Berg, 1971). Unexpectedly positive biopsy specimens have not been met with in Aberdeen. In 4 patients peroral jejunal biopsies did confirm the presence of Crohn's disease that had been suspected at earlier barium studies or laparotomy. Histological examination of biopsy specimens from 10 other patients showed no specific abnormality. However, the investigations were helpful in excluding conditions such as idiopathic steatorrhoea. Histochemical and microbiological studies are possible on capsule specimens.

Differential Diagnosis

As knowledge about and awareness of Crohn's disease increases, the percentage of correct diagnoses made at first consultation will increase. In the past it has been low, varying from 6 per cent (Dyer and Dawson, 1970) to 14 per cent (Fährlander and Baerlocher, 1971), even in centres interested in the disease. Table 1 sets out the conditions from which

Table 1

*Differential diagnosis of Crohn's disease
according to the presenting symptom*

1. Diarrhoea	ulcerative colitis, steatorrhoea, dysentery
2. Intestinal colic	mechanical obstruction carcinoma
3. Diarrhoea + colic	gastroenteritis, carcinoid syndrome
4. Pain + pyrexia	acute appendicitis, diverticulitis
5. Colic + mass	carcinoma, appendix abscess, reticulosis
6. Fistulae + mass	tuberculosis, actinomycosis
7. Pain in R.I.F.	chronic appendix, urological disease, endometriosis
8. Pyrexia of unknown origin	subacute bacterial endocarditis, rheumatic fever, brucellosis, reticulosis
9. Bleeding	carcinoma, polyp, diverticulum, proctitis, colitis

Crohn's disease must be differentiated acording to the presenting symptoms. In both the Basle and St Bartholomew's Hospital series an erroneous initial diagnosis of ulcerative colitis was made in 19 per cent of patients who were finally shown to have Crohn's disease. Appendicitis, with or without an abscess, was an almost equally common misdiagnosis. When the patient is over the age of 50 years cancer or diverticulitis are likely to be suspected. These diseases are considered in more detail below.

One group of patients who have received little attention are those who have acquired an enteric infection and have been unable to shake it off. It is increasingly common in Britain to have young women referred to an Out Patient Clinic in the autumn with a provisional diagnosis of Crohn's disease. They have been abroad during the summer holidays and contracted some form of gastroenteritis. Colicky abdominal pain and diarrhoea have persisted intermittently and 2–3 kg weight may have been lost during the same number of months. It is important in these patients to find out if any other member of their family or holiday party was affected and what treatment was given. Often several remedies have been tried, usually for an insufficient length of time. Culture of faeces is advisable but may not reveal any pathogenic bacteria. Radiological appearances are normal. An adequate course of oral neomycin or sulphaguanidine will usually cure the symptoms.

Patients must always be asked about residence abroad and whether they have had more serious enteric infections, for example typhoid fever, amoebic or bacillary dysentery. When these diseases are suspected, appropriate serological and faecal examinations are indicated. Abdominal tuberculosis is rare in Britain today, but it may appear in a patient who has spent part of his or her life in a less developed region of the world.

It is not possible to discuss all the diseases which may produce symptoms and signs similar to those that are caused by Crohn's disease. Recurrent urinary infection or ureteral obstruction may puzzle a urologist if he does not consider the possibility of inflammatory bowel disease. A pelvic mass in a female understandably is often regarded as an ovarian cyst, or if tender as salpingitis or tubo-ovarian abscess. An orthopaedic surgeon may treat a patient with ankylosing spondylitis long before any evidence of intestinal involvement appears.

The conditions from which Crohn's disease has most frequently to be differentiated are the following—

1. Ulcerative Colitis. Idiopathic ulcerative proctocolitis is several times more common than Crohn's disease. Patients are often young. The onset in ulcerative colitis is sometimes sudden and may be related to a psychological upset. Bowel movements are more frequent than in Crohn's disease. In colitis there may be 10–20 watery motions in 24 hours; in Crohn's disease the daily total is usually only half that number. Colicky pain is an almost invariable feature of Crohn's disease, while it is rare in ulcerative colitis (Lennard-Jones *et al.*, 1968). There is more loss of blood per rectum in the latter disease, but fissures and fistulae around the anus are much less common than in Crohn's disease. Remissions and relapses tend to be more dramatic in ulcerative colitis, when compared to the more slowly fluctuating and progressive course of Crohn's disease. A mass is present in less than one-half of all patients with Crohn's disease and is absent in ulcerative colitis. On sigmoidoscopy in colitis there is almost invariably a uniform mucosal inflammation of the rectum.

Radiologically the changes in ulcerative colitis are maximal on the left side of the colon and are in continuity. Crohn's disease often spares the distal colon and rectum; the lesions are discontinuous, with normal colon present between areas of ulceration and stenosis. A narrowed, rigid and ulcerated terminal ileum is diagnostic of Crohn's disease. There can be a "backwash ileitis" in ulcerative colitis; the lower ileum may be oedematous and irritable but is not rigid and stenosed—indeed it may appear slightly dilated. Symmetrical involvement of the circumference of the colon is the rule in ulcerative colitis, whereas the thickened patches of Crohn's disease for a time may appear asymmetrical. Pseudopolyp formation is commoner in ulcerative colitis, but the earlier mucosal oedema and ulceration may be seen in both diseases. The presence of a fistula strongly suggests that the diagnosis is Crohn's disease.

Histologically ulcerative colitis principally affects the mucosa (mucosal colitis). All layers of the bowel wall are infiltrated by inflammatory cells in Crohn's disease (transmural colitis). On rectal biopsy the disproportionate infiltration of the submucosa may be diagnostic of Crohn's disease even when granulomas and giant cells are not seen.

In any large series of patients with ulcerative bowel disease there are usually 10–15 per cent of cases where for some time it is not possible to say whether the lesion is ulcerative colitis or Crohn's disease. Repeated investigations and the gradual unfolding of the natural history of the disease over months or years usually allow a final diagnosis to be made.

2. Appendicitis. Most patients whose Crohn's disease mimics acute appendicitis are admitted to hospital as emergencies. The signs of acute peritoneal irritation in the right iliac fossa may make it seem inadvisable to wait and undertake elaborate tests. Instead laparotomy is performed. It may be unavoidable if a potentially fatal peritonitis from appendicitis is to be avoided and certainly it enables a competent surgeon to make an accurate diagnosis. However, if these patients are questioned carefully, some will admit to having had diarrhoea for a few days or at intervals in the past. Acute appendicitis usually only gives rise to diarrhoea at the extremes of life. Young babies very rarely get Crohn's disease. Old patients are liable to have colonic rather than ileal Crohn's disease, so that signs would not necessarily be maximal in the right lower abdomen. Fever and vomiting are less common in Crohn's disease than in genuine appendicitis and muscular guarding is less marked. While it is unlikely that there will be any occult blood in the faeces in acute appendicitis, in most cases there is a definite leucocytosis.

"Chronic appendicitis" is a somewhat doubtful entity. Faecoliths in the lumen or fibrosis in the wall of a normally situated (pelvic brim or retrocaecal) appendix will not produce diarrhoea or the radiological changes of Crohn's disease, although they may cause recurrent pain. When the appendix lies in the rare retro-ileal position the simulation may be much closer. The author has seen 2 patients with a faecolith or foreign-body in a retro-ileal appendix which apparently was causing mild diarrhoea and a persistent deformity of the terminal ileum on barium enema examination.

3. Cancer. Sarcoma of the small intestine is rare. Initially a leiomyosarcoma tends to grow outward and not encroach on the lumen. It finally presents as either a mass or intestinal haemorrhage. Lymphosarcoma can mimic Crohn's disease and give rise to diarrhoea. The centre of the tumour is often excavated, so that there is relatively little interference with the passage of intestinal contents. On radiological screening a mass is felt at the site of mucosal disorganization and destruction. The mass is unlikely to be tender and the ileal lumen is dilated rather than stenosed. The lesion is an isolated one and other loops of intestine are not splayed apart by mesenteric thickening.

Very occasionally a patient with a malignant reticulosis such as Hodgkin's disease will have multiple lesions in the small intestine. There is likely to be other evidence of the condition, for example in the cervical nodes and enlarged spleen. Radiologically several stenosed areas are detected; in one or two sites the abnormality may be eccenteric or a projecting mass may be demonstrated (Linden and Marshak, 1970).

Carcinoma of the large intestine is very much more common than its ileal counterpart. Patients are usually over the age of 50 years and the history is only of a few months' duration. Crohn's disease of the colon in general causes a persistent type of diarrhoea. With cancer of the colon short bouts of diarrhoea alternate with longer periods of constipation. Even when looseness of the bowels continues for months and no organic lesion can be demonstrated, it is extremely unlikely that a malignant neoplasm is responsible (Hawkins and Cockel, 1971).

There is no pyrexia and external fistulae and skip lesions do not develop in patients with colonic cancer. Barium enema examinations give good definition of these neoplasms. Typically there is a single lesion, with shouldering effect at its ends, and mucosal destruction within the short affected segment. On the proximal side there is often dilatation of the bowel. More than half of all intestinal cancers are in the distal sigmoid colon or rectum, and consequently are within easy reach of an endoscope. Unfortunately, cancer in the caecum or ascending colon often has an insidious onset and is not accessible for biopsy examination. A few such neoplasms develop in patients under 30 years of age. In malignant disease time will always reveal the error in diagnosis. However, if the patient is to be given a chance of survival, laparotomy is essential when, after reasonably rapid investigation, there is any remaining possibility of cancer being present.

4. Diverticulitis. Both peridiverticulitis and Crohn's disease occur in older patients. By chance they must frequently co-exist, as diverticulosis is common in the elderly. The high roughage diet prescribed for diverticular disease would worsen the pain and discomfort of a patient with transmural colitis. Pain and fever are more severe and noticeable in diverticulitis than in Crohn's disease. The reverse is true for diarrhoea and rectal bleeding (Schmidt *et al.*, 1968) although uninflamed colonic diverticula sometimes cause brisk haemorrhage. In their early stages the radiological changes seen in the two conditions may be difficult to differentiate from each other, particularly when Crohn's disease takes the form of an isolated lesion. The rose-thorn fissures or spicules of Crohn's disease are up to 3 mm deep and unevenly spaced; they progress to form fistulae. The serrations of early diverticulosis are less deep and more regular, but eventually expand into retort-shaped pulsion diverticulae.

When there are recurrent perianal fistulae and fissures, with oedematous, discoloured skin, the underlying pathological process is almost certainly Crohn's disease. A rectal biopsy will probably prove diagnostic.

5. Ischaemic Colitis. This rare vascular abnormality generally affects the left side of the colon, usually in patients more than 50 years old (Marston *et al.*, 1966). Some patients have hypertension, a collagen disease, or evidence of peripheral vascular insufficiency. As in other parts of the body atherosclerosis, emboli, thrombosis or trauma obviously can interrupt the arterial supply to the colon. However, in most cases the aetiology is not known. Selective mesenteric angiograms show the main arteries to the transverse and descending colons to be patent. It has been postulated that there is a transient spasm of blood vessels of arteriolar size, the ischaemia being sufficient to damage all coats of the colon wall, especially in the vicinity of the splenic flexure. It has been suggested that there may be a low flow state or splanchnic vasoconstriction due to excessive production of noradrenaline. The contraceptive pill has also been blamed. Subsequent infection from staphylococci or *Cl. Welchii* in the gut lumen is said to produce the condition known as pseudo-enterocolitis, with necrosis and membrane formation. A great deal of study and explanation about the aetiology of this form of vascular brinkmanship are required. Various forms of intravascular coagulation merit investigation.

The typical clinical history is said to be of an elderly patient who is suddenly seized by left upper abdominal pain. Later some blood may be passed per rectum—bleeding is not normally associated with the interruption of the blood supply. There seems to be a tendency for ischaemic colitis to undergo spontaneous resolution. There is often diarrhoea and maybe tenesmus. During the first day or two a barium enema shows a coarse cobblestone or thumb-printing appearance in the colon, not unlike that of Crohn's disease. Fibrous tissue laid down in the damaged wall begins to contract, and a short smooth stricture results in the majority of patients. It would be most unusual for Crohn's disease of the colon to have such a sudden and bloody presentation.

6. Tuberculosis. One of the popular misconceptions about tuberculous enteritis and colitis is that there is open, pulmonary disease. In fact the chest X-ray is very often normal (Schuster, 1971). The patients notice considerable lassitude, sweating is troublesome at night, and there is irregular pyrexia. In the earlier stages there is diarrhoea. Later, with attempted healing, multiple strictures appear in the intestine. Because of the stagnation that tight strictures produce, there is malabsorption and a megaloblastic anaemia may develop. Straight X-ray of the abdomen mostly shows calcification in lymph nodes or other structures. Unfortunately this finding by no means excludes Crohn's disease. Histological and microbiological study of a resected mass often is necessary in order to substantiate the diagnosis of hypertrophic ileo-caecal tuberculosis (Anscombe *et al.*, 1967). Caseation is present and acid-fast bacilli may be seen—it is advisable to culture them and carry out guinea-pig inoculations to be certain the bacilli are *My. tuberculosis.*

7. Other Conditions. *Jejunal diverticula* usually appear in elderly subjects. Some are symptomless. Other patients have abdominal discomfort, flatulence and anorexia. Bacterial proliferation can give rise to severe steatorrhoea and defective vitamin B_{12} absorption (Cooke *et al.*, 1963). The diverticula are shown up on a barium meal; there may be some doubt as to whether they are primary or are secondary to skip lesions of Crohn's disease. However, the ileum looks normal. Patients with Crohn's disease are mostly young.

Several chemicals, notably potassium chloride tablets, have been incriminated in the causation of *small intestinal ulcers* (Davies and Brightmore, 1970). Enquiry must be made about any drugs taken in the recent past. *Eosinophilic infiltration* of the gastro-intestinal tract can simulate Crohn's disease, but the marked eosinophilia which many of the patients have should give a clue to the real diagnosis (O'Neill, 1970). A *stenosing type of jejunitis* has been described by Aubrey (1971). There is intermittent diarrhoea and a feeling of distension. The exact relationship between stenosing jejunitis and both Crohn's disease and simple jejunal ulcers at present is uncertain.

Endometriosis of the intestine is always a possibility in women during the reproductive phase of life. In 9 cases out of 10 it is the colon rather than the ileum that is involved (Macafee and Greer, 1960). There is colicky abdominal pain, vomiting and distension at the time of menstruation. Obstruction may supervene. In most patients laparoscopy reveals other evidence of endometriosis in the pelvis.

One iatrogenic disease of the intestine, *radiation enteritis*, clinically is virtually indistinguishable from Crohn's disease (Tankel *et al.*, 1965; De Crosse *et al.*, 1969). The previous history is all-important. Radiotherapy for genital tract cancer in women is the commonest cause; nearly 12 per cent of such patients get some intestinal symptoms, with diarrhoea proceeding later on to stricture formation. Ankylosing spondylitis may have been the reason for giving irradiation treatment. The intestinal injuries tend to be multiple. Fat, xylose and vitamin B_{12}

absorption are commonly impaired after 1–2 years. Fistulae appear and as in Crohn's disease they do not respond to conservative treatment.

References

Anderson, F. H. and Bogoch, A. (1968), *Canad. med. Ass. J.*, **98**, 150.
Anscombe, A. R., Keddie, N. C. and Schofield, P. F. (1967), *Gut*, **8**, 337.
Atwell, J. D. (1964), *Gastroenterology*, **46**, 16.
Aubrey, D. A. (1971), *Brit. J. Surg.*, **58**, 633.
Badley, B. W. D., Murphy, G. M. and Bouchier, I. A. D. (1969), *Lancet*, **2**, 400.
Beeken, W. L. (1969), *Gastroenterology*, **56**, 1138.
Bendixen, G., Jarnum, S., Soltoft, J., Westergaard, H., Weeke, B. and Yssing, M. (1968), *Scand. J. Gastroent.*, **3**, 481.
Berg, N. O. (1971), *Acta Paediat. Scand.*, **60**, 105.
Best, C. N. (1959), *Brit. med. J.*, **2**, 862.
Booth, C. C., Hanna, S., Babouris, N. and McIntyre, I. (1963), *Brit. med. J.*, **2**, 141.
Brahme, F. and Lindstrom, C. (1970), *Gut*, **11**, 928.
Brahme, F. and Wenckert, A. (1970), *Gut*, **11**, 576.
Brahme, F. (1971), in *Regional Enteritis* (*Crohn's Disease*). Eds. A. Enkel and T. Larsson, p. 81. Stockholm: Skandia International Symposia.
Capek, V., Maratka, Z., Kubernatova, D. and Kudrmann, J. (1968), *Cs. Gastroent. Vyz.*, **22**, 254.
Chalfin, D. and Holt, P. R. (1968), *Amer. J. Dig. Dis.*, **12**, 81.
Chanarin, I. and Bennett, M. C. (1962), *Brit. med. J.*, **1**, 985.
Cooke, W. T. (1955), *Ann. R. Coll. Surg. Engl.*, **17**, 137.
Cooke, W. T., Cox, E. V., Fone, D. J., Meynell, M. J. and Gaddie, R. (1963), *Gut*, **4**, 115.
Cooke, W. T., Fowler, D. J., Cox, E. V., Gaddie, R. and Meynell, M. J. (1958), *Gastroenterology*, **34**, 910.
Cox, E. V., Meynell, M. J., Cooke, W. T. and Gaddie, R. (1958), *Gastroenterology*, **35**, 390.
Cummack, D. H. (1969), *Gastro-Intestinal X-ray Diagnosis, A Descriptive Atlas*. p. 126. Edinburgh and London: E. & S. Livingstone.
Davies, D. R. and Brightmore, T. (1970), *Brit. J. Surg.*, **57**, 134.
Dean, A. C. B. and Shearman, D. J. C. (1970), *Lancet*, **1**, 550.
De Cosse, J. J., Rhodes, R., Wentz, W. B., Reagan, J. W., Dworken, H. J. and Holden, W. D. (1969), *Ann. Surg.*, **170**, 369.
Dick, A. P., Lennard-Jones, J. E., Jones, J. H. and Morson, B. C. (1970), *Gut*, **11**, 182.
Dotevall, G. and Kock, N. G. (1968), *Scand. J. Gastroent.*, **3**, 293.
Dyer, N. H., Rutherford, C., Visick, J. H. and Dawson, A. M. (1970), *Brit. J. Radiol.*, **43**, 401.
Dyer, N. H. and Dawson, A. M. (1971), *Scand. J. Gastroent.*, **6**, 253.
Eklöf, O. and Gierup, H. J. W. (1970), *Amer. J. Roentgenol.*, **108**, 624.
Fahrländer, H. and Baerlocher, C. (1971), in *Regional Enteritis* (*Crohn's Disease*). Eds. A. Engel and T. Larsson, p. 131. Stockholm: Skandia International Symposia.
Fielding, J. F. (1971), *J. Irish med. Assoc.*, **64**, 221.
Fielding, J. F., Cooke, W. T. and Williams, J. A. (1971), *Lancet*, **1**, 1106.
Filipe, M. I. and Dawson, I. (1970), *Gut*, **11**, 229.
Fone, D. J., Cooke, W. T., Meynell, M. J. and Harris, E. L. (1961), *Gut*, **2**, 218.
Friedenberg, M. J., McAlister, W. H. and Margulis, A. R. (1962), *Amer. J. Roentgenol.*, **88**, 693.
Fry, I. K. and Stanley, P. (1971), *Proc. Roy. Soc. Med.*, **64**, 171.
Gerlach, K. (1970), *Gastroenterology*, **59**, 567.

Gudmand-Hoyer, E. and Jarnum, S. (1970), *Gut*, **11**, 338.
Hansing, B. and Meeuwisse, G. (1971), *Acta Paediat. Scand.*, **60**, 104.
Harrer, W. V., Goldstein, F. and Wirts, C. W. (1970), *Gastroenterology*, **59**, 862.
Harris, O. D., Philip, H. M., Cooke, W. T. and Power, W. F. R. (1970), *Scand. J. Gastroent.*, **5**, 169.
Hawkins, C. F. and Cockel, R. (1971), *Gut*, **12**, 208.
Head, L. H., Heaton, J. W. and Kivel, R. M. (1969), *Gastroenterology*, **56**, 571.
Heaton, F. W. (1967), *Brit. J. Surg.*, **54**, 41.
Hermos, J. A., Cooper, H. L., Kramer, P. and Trier, J. S. (1970), *Gastroenterology*, **59**, 868.
Hoffbrand, A. V., Stewart, J. S., Booth, C. C. and Mollin, D. (1968), *Brit. med. J.*, **2**, 71.
Jackson, B. B. (1958), *Ann. Surg.*, **148**, 81.
Jones, J. H., Lennard-Jones, J. E. and Young, A. C. (1969), *Gut*, **10**, 738.
Kantor, J. L. (1934), *J. Amer. med. Ass.*, **103**, 2016.
Krause, U., Bergman, L. and Norlen, B. J. (1971), *Scand. J. Gastroent.*, **6**, 97.
Kyle, J. (1971), *Scot. med. J.*, **16**, 197.
Lennard-Jones, J. E., Lockhart-Mummery, H. E. and Morson, B. C. (1968), *Gastroenterology*, **54**, 1162.
Lennard-Jones, J. E. (1971), *Proc. Roy. Soc. Med.*, **64**, 177.
Lockhart-Mummery, H. E. and Morson, B. C. (1964), *Gut*, **5**, 493.
Lunderquist, A. and Knutsson, H. (1967), *Amer. J. Roentg.*, **101**, 338.
Macafee, C. H. G. and Greer, H. L. H. (1960), *J. Obstet. Gynec. Br. Commonwealth*, **67**, 539.
Marshak, R. H. and Linder, A. E. (1970), *Radiology of the Small Intestine*, p. 158. Philadelphia and London: W. B. Saunders.
Marston, A., Pheils, M. T. and Morson, B. C. (1966), *Gut*, **7**, 1.
Morowitz, D. A. (1968), *Ann. Intern. Med.*, **68**, 1013.
Morson, B. C. (1971), "Hurst Memorial Lecture", Newcastle-upon-Tyne.
Nagasako, K., Yazawa, C. and Takemoto, T. (1971), *Gastroenterology*, **60**, 823.
Nygaard, K., Helsingen, N. and Rootwelt, K. (1970), *Scand. J. Gastroent.*, **5**, 349.
O'Neill, T. (1970), *Brit. J. Surg.*, **57**, 704.
Pimparkar, B. D., Mouhran, Y. and Bockus, H. (1960), *Proc. Internat. Congress Gastroent.*, Leiden, p. 227.
Potocky, V., Balcar, V. and Setka, J. (1968), *Cs. Gastroent. Vyz.*, **22**, 263.
Present, D. H., Chapman, M. L., Cohen, N. and Janowitz, H. D. (1967), *Gastroenterology*, **53**, 1113.
Salmon, P. R., Branch, R. A., Collins, C., Espiner, H. and Read, A. E. (1971), *Gut*, **12**, 729.
Schmidt, G. T., Lennard-Jones, J. E., Morson, B. C. and Young, A. C. (1968), *Gut*, **9**, 7.
Schofield, P. F. (1967), *Dis. Colon Rect.*, **10**, 262.
Schuster, M. M. (1971), *Gastroenterology*, **60**, 715.
Smith, A. N. (1971), in *Regional Enteritis (Crohn's Disease)*. Eds. A. Engel and T. Larsson, p. 41. Stockholm: Skandia International Symposia.
Smith, M. P. (1967), *J. Amer. med. Ass.*, **201**, 890.
Steinberg, F. (1961), *New Engl. J. Med.*, **264**, 186.
Steinfeld, J. L., Davidson, J. D., Gordon, R. S. and Greene, F. B. (1960), *Amer. J. Med.*, **29**, 405.
Tankel, H. I., Clark, D. H. and Lee, F. D. (1965), *Gut*, **6**, 560.
Tygat, G., Vantrappen, G., Rutgeerts, L. and Vandenbroucke, J. (1967), *Acta Chir. Belg. Suppl.*, **2**, 66.
Weeke, B. and Jarnum, S. (1971), *Gut*, **12**, 297.

Chapter VII
Complications

There is no simple definition of what constitutes a complication in Crohn's disease. A few patients do suffer from some epiphenomenon superimposed on a straightforward and well localized lesion, for example perforation or haemorrhage. Far more often after a number of years the ill-effects of chronic disease and of unsuccessful attempts at treatment become hopelessly interlinked and cannot be clearly separated from each other. This is true in many advanced cases with malnutrition and subacute obstruction. Time of appearance cannot be used to separate complications from ordinary clinical features because ankylosing spondylitis and fistula-in-ano are liable to be present for years before there is any evidence of Crohn's disease in the intestine. Unusual, late or unexpected developments are grouped together here as "complications" and may be classified as local or general. In the following pages they are considered in approximately the order of their importance in clinical practice.

Intestinal Obstruction

The transmural nature of the lesion even in early Crohn's disease causes some interference with the normal onward propulsive movements of the intestine. In this sense there is some element of obstruction in many cases of Crohn's disease. Irritation of the wall expedites the passage of intestinal contents, but spasm may temporarily arrest their progress. Later on the gradual contraction of fibrous tissue in the damaged wall narrows the lumen and eventually the stenosis presents a formidable mechanical obstruction. The fluid contents of the ileum can pass through a comparatively small lumen. However, increasingly powerful peristalsis is required to overcome the obstruction, and this gives rise to severe, colicky abdominal pain, which is a common feature of Crohn's disease.

When peristaltic activity is only partially successful, the intestine proximal to the stenosed segment becomes progressively dilated. Clinically it is recognized that the patient has developed the complication of subacute obstruction. The abdomen is moderately distended, loud bowel sounds are audible and if the patient is emaciated, visible peristalsis may be seen. Vomiting is not as common as in some other types of small intestinal obstruction. The patient nearly always continues to pass loose stools, although the total faecal volume per 24 hours is decreased.

It is most uncommon for obstruction to become complete, with absolute constipation. There was only one case out of 175 in Aberdeen that could have been considered as having complete obstruction, and with more persistence the transient obstruction might have been overcome by non-operative means. In a survey of small intestinal obstruction in Cincinatti, Neely (1962) had 4 cases due to Crohn's disease out of a series of 346 adults with acute obstruction. This incidence of slightly more than 1 per cent is the usual experience in general hospitals. Recently Davis and Sperling (1969) in Los Angeles blamed Crohn's disease for blocking the bowel in 6 out of 165 patients, but the obstruction may sometimes have been subacute. Other complications, such as abscess formation and adhesions from earlier operations, may of course produce complete mechanical obstruction. Five per cent of primary operations for Crohn's disease in Leeds were carried out on account of obstruction; this indication was 3 times more common among those requiring further surgery (de Dombal *et al.*, 1971), almost certainly because of adhesions and other sequelae of the first laparotomy.

When the patient is known to have Crohn's disease the treatment of subacute obstruction is by nasogastric aspiration and administration of intravenous fluid and electrolytes. The more distressing symptoms subside and with a period of intensive medical therapy (page 157) the patient can be made fit for elective surgery. Some patients are admitted to hospital with obstructive signs but without any previous investigations or diagnosis. Straight X-ray of the abdomen (page 89) shows some distended loops of bowel, and with tenderness present in the lower abdomen, some type of internal strangulated hernia may be suspected and laparotomy carried out. In these circumstances and if obstruction is not complete, unless the surgeon is experienced, it may be safer to close the abdomen and treat the patient conservatively. A short-circuiting procedure is necessary when obstruction is complete, but the recurrence rate of Crohn's disease is high if the diseased segment is not excluded from the faecal stream.

Malabsorption

There is always liable to be some impairment of absorption of foodstuffs in Crohn's disease. The majority of patients have lost weight when they are first seen. When the loss exceeds 10 kg, and particularly when it continues after the institution of medical therapy, it becomes a matter of major concern. The severely malnourished patient generally is one of the small number of unfortunate people in whom Crohn's disease has progressed over many years in spite of multiple operations. He looks emaciated and haggard. His cheeks are sunken, the conjunctivae are pale, and stomatitis and cheilosis may be present. The limbs are reduced to skin and bone, the skin frequently having a scaly surface and showing irregular pigmentation. With hypo-albuminaemia there is dependent oedema. In contrast to the match-like limbs, sub-acute obstruction or steatorrhoea cause abdominal distension; one or more external fistulae may be obvious on the scarred abdomen. Bor-borygmi are audible, visible peristalsis may be seen and on percussion there is a tympanitic note. A child will show stunting of growth and a young woman will have secondary amenorrhoea.

Malnutrition may result from inadequate calorie intake with normal absorption, from high intake with severe malabsorption or from the increased catabolism associated with sepsis and fistulae (Clark and Lauder, 1969). Deficient intake may be due to faulty dietary habits or more often to anorexia or the fear that eating will produce pain. Co-operation with a dietitian is essential to ensure that the diet is correct. An intake of over 3,000 calories per day should be aimed at (see page 150). Corticosteroids not uncommonly improve the appetite, but increase catabolism. Surgical intervention may be necessary to prevent post-prandial colic and for the proper drainage of abscesses.

Most severely malnourished patients have marked defects in absorp-tion, usually resulting from a combination of factors. The small intestinal mucosa is diseased, the lower ileum may have been resected and there is a break in the normally almost closed recycling system for bile salts. Pancreatic exocrine function remains remarkably good after operations for Crohn's disease (Petersen *et al.*, 1969). Fat absorption suffers most when the ileum is diseased: there may be 10–20 gm of fat lost in the faeces each day. With this degree of steatorrhoea, deficiences of fat-soluble vitamins A, D and K may gradually appear, and excessive amounts of magnesium and calcium are lost from the body. Malabsorp-tion of fat, vitamins A and B_{12} is more frequent after resections for ileal disease than after colectomy (Hertzberg *et al.*, 1969). Replacement therapy must be carried out energetically and with enthusiasm by all concerned in order to fully correct the numerous deficiencies that may be present. There is some evidence that adaptation of vitamin B_{12} absorption may take place 3–12 months after ileal bypass surgery (Nygaard *et al.*, 1970).

The hypochronic anaemia of Crohn's disease is accounted for almost entirely by bleeding from the ulcerated mucosa into the gut lumen. A healthy man excretes 1 mg/day of iron in the faeces, equivalent to shedding 2 ml of blood. Menstruation doubles the normal daily loss in women. When the faecal occult blood test is positive it means that at least 5 ml of blood have entered the gut. Larger amounts are likely to be lost in Crohn's disease, with consequent depletion of the body's reserves of iron. The red bone marrow's ability to respond to anaemia is impaired when the plasma iron level falls below 70 μg/100 ml (Hillman and Henderson, 1969). With chronic inflammation available iron may have difficulty in reaching the marrow. The red cells become smaller in size (MCV), followed by a decrease in the amount of haemoglobin they contain (MCH) and in the mean cell haemoglobin concentration (MCHC). With the persistent loss of iron into the gut in long-standing Crohn's disease, the haemoglobin concentration in severe cases may fall to 8 gm per 100 ml, or less. The anaemia mostly responds to oral ferrous sulphate. If major surgery is contemplated within a few days, transfusion of packed red cells is desirable.

Folate acts as a co-enzyme in many forms of protein synthesis. Adequate amounts are present in a good mixed diet but unfortunately folate is readily destroyed, for example by sunlight, pasteurization and cooking. In many patients with Crohn's disease the folate deficiency is probably the result of inadequate intake. Sufficient vitamin B_{12}-intrinsic factor complex for normal red cell formation usually reaches the ileum of patients. When there has been an extensive resection of diseased ileum, vitamin B_{12} uptake is markedly impaired. Bacterial proliferation in areas of stasis, blind loops and diverticulae can reduce the amount of B_{12} available for absorption, although folate may be manufactured in such situations (Hoffbrand *et al.*, 1971). In any of these patients macrocytic anaemia gradually develops. The first indication is an increase in the mean red cell volume (MCV). Later variations in the size of the red cells and a neutropenia are discernible on the film. Only a small number of patients with Crohn's disease in practice develop macrocytic anaemia, but a regular check should be kept on the MCV of patients during long-term surveillance.

Protein absorption is likely to be normal unless there is widespread jejuno-ileal disease. However, the nitrogen output in the faeces and urine may rise, this loss being consequent upon the catabolic stimulus provided by infection. Much of the nitrogen comes from the breakdown of protein in muscle. The discharge from external fistulae does not in itself contribute significantly to the nitrogen loss, but eradication of associated infection will assist the patient to return to a positive nitrogen balance.

Carbohydrate absorption is not interfered with until most of the small intestine has been excised. When only 90 cm remain, there may be lactose intolerance (Richards *et al.*, 1971). There can be no justification for pushing resection to such an extreme that the patient is left with a crippling short bowel syndrome (Melich, 1969).

Fistula Formation

One of the best known and most feared complications of Crohn's disease is the formation of a fistula. The reported overall incidence varies from 30–40 per cent, but with better understanding and experience of the disease the incidence met with under older methods of management should decrease in the future.

There are 3 types of fistulae—internal, external and ano-rectal. An internal fistula is truly spontaneous. It is the outcome of one or more fissures which have penetrated right through the bowel wall and perhaps formed a small, silent, extramural abscess (the "closed perforation" of American usage). Eventually it reaches and discharges into an adjacent loop of ileum or other viscus, forming a somewhat indirect fistula

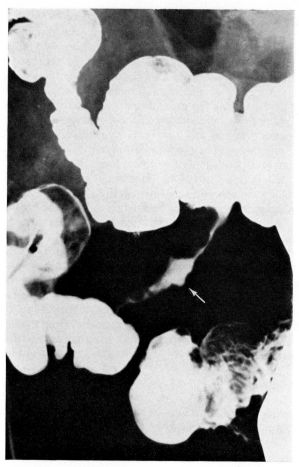

Fig. 1. Internal fistula. The indirect track demonstrated on barium enema examination passes through a small abscess cavity (arrow).

(Fig. 1). An external fistula to the anterior abdominal wall nearly always follows an operative procedure, and comes out through the incision; fistulae to the umbilicus have been described (Hiley *et al.*, 1971). The author restricts the use of the term "ano-rectal fistula" to those cases where a complete fistulous tract has been demonstrated; perianal abscesses, etc., are not included if a fistula is only suspected.

The respective incidences of these fistulae in 6 large series from North America and Britain are shown in Table 1. A patient may have more than one type of fistula, the most frequent combination in Aberdeen being external and ano-rectal fistulae.

Table 1

Incidence of fistulae in Crohn's disease

Series	Region	Fistulae (*per cent*)		
		Internal	*External*	*Ano-rectal*
Van Patter *et al*. (1954)	Mayo Clinic	14	10	31
Crohn and Yarnis (1958)	New York	16	10	14
Edwards (1964)	London	11	8	19
Schofield (1965)	Manchester	10	12	20
Perrett *et al*. (1971)	Oxford	12	14	—
Kyle (1971)	Aberdeen	9	14	10

Internal Fistulae. Frequently an internal fistula between loops of bowel is not suspected until it is revealed by barium studies or at operation. There may be several fistulae, most often between adjacent parts of the ileum but occasionally opening into the transverse colon. Considering the proximity of the sigmoid loop to the terminal ileum, it is surprising that ileo-sigmoid fistulae are not established. There are only 3 reports in the literature, where in patients with severe disease a complex communication between ileum, sigmoid and bladder finally developed (Pugh, 1945; Mellin, 1959; Cornet *et al*., 1963). Because most interintestinal fistulae are narrow and tortuous they do not themselves significantly reduce transit time or lead to profuse diarrhoea. A direct ileo-sigmoid fistula could have serious consequences. A duodenosigmoid fistula following pregnancy has been described (Holzback and Jones, 1969).

When diseased ileum lies in the bottom of the pelvis it may be in contact with the bladder or vault of the vagina, and give rise to repeated cystitis and cervicitis. A fissure after making its way through the thickened ileal wall insidiously creates an ileo-vesical or ileo-vaginal fistula.

Ileo-vesical Fistula. Crohn's disease is responsible for only 4 per cent of all entero-vesical fistulae, but for no less than 40 per cent of those between the ileum and the urinary bladder. There were 97 bladder fistulae complicating Crohn's disease in the literature up to the end of 1967. Kyle and Murray (1969) added 10 more cases. All these 10 patients had an intractable form of Crohn's disease, symptoms of which had been present for a mean interval of 5·5 years before detection of the fistula. Males were more often affected than females, and with one 70 year old exception, the patients were comparatively young. Frequency and dysuria were experienced by half the patients for some months, before pneumaturia was noticed. Strangury was very distressing for 2 patients but haematuria occurred only once. Pneumaturia is a dramatic symptom for any patient, but it was not part of the initial presentation in any of the 10 cases. Since 1969, one more case has been seen in Aberdeen. This was a 70 year old man whose first complaint was pneumaturia. Numerous investigations and a period of observation in hospital failed to substantiate his story. However, he at last proved it most convincingly by passing faecal material per urethram around an indwelling Foley catheter!

Cystoscopy in each of the 10 patients revealed a reddened, oedematous area on the postero-lateral bladder wall. Injections of air, dye and contrast media through rectum or bladder failed to demonstrate the fistula, and pyelography was normal. When flatus and, less often, faeces are reaching the bladder, operation is necessary. Resection of affected ileum is the treatment of choice. The opening in the bladder is difficult to find on the peritoneal surface and the surgeon may have to be content with oversewing and draining the area.

Ileo-vaginal Fistula. Women suffer from Crohn's disease more frequently than do men, yet only 11 cases of fistula into the vagina had been recorded by 1969. In that year Kyle and Sinclair described a 21 year old woman, known to have Crohn's disease, who developed an offensive, irritating vaginal discharge. A short-circuit with exclusion has cured all her symptoms, except that she remains infertile. A second gravely ill female, aged 28 years, was also diagnosed as having an ileo-vaginal fistula. It appeared half way through a succession of operations that were undertaken in a vain bid to cure the Crohn's disease from which she died. Mathews *et al.* (1971) have added 2 more examples from Texas, bringing the total number of cases with ileo-vaginal fistulae to 15.

Recto-vaginal fistula allegedly is not uncommon. Van Patter *et al.* (1954) had 10 fistulae of this type among 266 females with all forms of Crohn's disease. The incidence is said to be considerably higher when colon and rectum are affected (Cornes and Stecher, 1961). No definite recto-vaginal fistula has been detected in the Aberdeen survey.

External Fistula. One-quarter of all external small bowel fistulae are caused by Crohn's disease (Lorenzo and Beal, 1969; Sheldon *et al.*, 1971). There were 25 such fistulae in the clinical series of 175 patients in Aberdeen. This incidence is disappointingly high. Three patients had suffered a partial breakdown of an anastomosis, 2 being specially referred for this reason from other parts of Scotland. In 4 cases drainage of an abscess in the right iliac fossa, thought to be the result of appendicitis, was followed by a persistent fistula. It is difficult to determine the precise cause of the external fistula in the remaining 18 patients, most of whom were treated before 1960. Prophylactic appendicectomy did not appear to be responsible. The reported incidence of fistula formation after appendicectomy varies from zero (Atwell *et al.*, 1966) to 30 per cent (Helms and Bradshaw, 1964). When the caecal wall is healthy the appendix can be safely removed. However, if Crohn's disease has spread to the caecum, the risk of fistula formation is increased. The fistula does not necessarily arise from the appendix stump; the point of origin is more likely to be located on the diseased ileal or caeca wall. Attempting to take a biopsy from unhealthy ileum is unwise.

Excoriation and digestion of the skin around an external fistula is rare except in those cases where there has been breakdown of an anastomosis. With profuse leakage, the fistula is acting as an unintended and uncontrolled ileostomy. Its surgical correction is clearly a matter of urgency. Much more frequently there is only a slight or intermittent mucopurulent discharge from an external fistula. The patient will often state that he feels less pain and distension when the fistula is open than when it is dry. Granulation tissue forms at the external orifice, and the surrounding skin is relatively intact.

It is advisable to outline the fistulous tract and its ramifications by fistulography. This is not always successful. While the presence of a small, persistent fistula strengthens the case for elective resection in Crohn's disease, it does not constitute an absolute indication for surgery. Local treatment to the external orifice of the fistula is useless.

Ano-rectal Fistula. Recurrent ano-rectal fistulae may be troublesome long before pain, diarrhoea and weight loss become manifest (Scharf, 1969). They develop again during the course of established Crohn's disease, their incidence rising the nearer the lower limit of the disease is to the anus. However, to get anal fistulae and Crohn's disease in the correct perspective, it is worth noting that Mazier (1971) found inflammatory bowel disease responsible for only 13 out of over 1,000 fistulae.

To insert a probe the whole way along the track of an ano-rectal fistula can be difficult. Almost certainly the 10 per cent incidence among Scottish patients is an under-estimate. On several occasions a fistula was suspected but could not be demonstrated in patients getting recurrent perianal or ischiorectal abscesses. Other workers may include such cases in their figures. A few unlucky patients do have very complex fistulae, with horse-shoe configuration and multiple orifices. The fistulae may extend far forward into the labia or neck of the scrotum.

When an abscess forms it requires to be laid open. Excision of a fistulous track provides material for histological examination and, for a time, relieves the patient of the annoyance of a perineal discharge. A permanent cure will not be achieved until the Crohn's disease higher up in the bowel has been eradicated. With colo-rectal disease this may mean procto-colectomy; faecal diversion by ileostomy or colostomy does not ensure disappearance of ano-rectal sepsis.

One Aberdeen patient has had a superior pelvirectal fistula for over 3 years. It apparently arises in ileum and tracks down through levator ani muscle, to open in the lateral part of the ischiorectal fossa. This patient presented more than 15 years ago with a pyrexia of unknown origin and has had several operations for recurrent disease. He has to wear a perineal pad, but in spite of this and numerous potential deficiencies, he continues to work every day. He exemplifies the fortitude displayed by many patients with chronic Crohn's disease.

Abscess

A large abscess may appear at some time in 20 per cent of patients with chronic Crohn's disease. Excluding minor wound infections and small recurrent abscesses on the anal margin, there were 35 major abscesses among 175 patients with Crohn's disease in the Aberdeen region. More than half these abscesses were in patients who developed internal or external fistulae. There were 9 large ischiorectal abscesses, some of them in patients who also had intra-abdominal suppuration. Five lower abdominal masses were at first thought to be appendix abscesses. In 15 patients the abscess appeared either shortly after an operation and in its immediate environs, or else close to an intestinal segment showing the changes of recurrent Crohn's disease. There were only 2 abscesses in the subphrenic spaces and in the liver. In 2 patients there had been bacterial inflammation in mesenteric nodes which had progressed to pus formation; this type of mesenteric abscess has been described previously (Rampai, 1963).

Most abscesses give rise to a swinging pyrexia and some may obstruct the intestine. Once an abscess is diagnosed it requires drainage urgently. The antibiotic sensitivity of the causative bacteria is determined. Thereafter the patient is prepared carefully for definitive surgery, which is undertaken when the patient is fit and local infection has been overcome.

Psoas Abscess. One of the more interesting complications recently recognized in Crohn's disease is a psoas abscess, a condition which at one time would have been regarded as pathognomonic of spinal tuberculosis. The large right ilio-psoas muscle lies directly behind the terminal ileum, while the left muscle has jejunum and sigmoid colon as anterior relations. Any fissure in ulcerated intestine which penetrates backwards rather than forwards or downwards should enter the psoas sheath. From there the abnormal channel will be able to track down towards the insertion of the muscle on the lesser trochanter of the femur. A straight X-ray of the hip may reveal a gas shadow lying in front of the joint capsule. During the 15 years up to the end of 1969, there were 4 patients with psoas abscess complicating Crohn's disease in north-east Scotland, and a fifth patient was specially referred to Aberdeen (Kyle, 1971). Brief details are given in Table 2. During the same period only 3 tuberculous psoas abscesses were seen. The second patient had had symptoms from extensive Crohn's enterocolitis for 11 years before she started to limp with her right leg. The fistula originated in a recurrence at the site of an earlier ileo-rectal anastomosis. By way of contrast the left hip flexion deformity and limp in the third patient

Table 2

Psoas abscess in Crohn's disease

Sex	Age at onset (years)	Presentation of abscess	Therapy	Result
M	13	L. groin swelling	Drainage, chemotherapy	Fair
F	15	Pain R. leg; limp	Ileo-proctocolectomy	Well
F	15	Flexed L. hip; pain	Drainage, steroids	Fair
M	29	R. groin swelling; pain	Resection	Recurrence
F	54	Pain and flexion R. hip	Drainage, steroids	Well

were part of the initial presentation of Crohn's disease. Three patients are still being maintained on medical treatment. The follow-up period is short and the possibility of these patients requiring resection at some time has not been ruled out.

Hepatic Changes in Crohn's Disease

All the portal blood draining from the small and large intestine passes through the liver which in consequence might be expected to show evidence of damage by blood-borne bacteria, toxins or breakdown. products released in the course of chronic inflammatory bowel disease- In addition gross malnutrition itself impairs hepatic cell function. Therefore it is surprising that in Crohn's disease the liver sometimes is undamaged. Until 1970 there were only a few reports on the state of the liver, their scarcity implying that liver disease did not constitute an obvious clinical problem. The small number of patients studied had often been highly selected—by death. Recently the results have been published of detailed examination of liver biopsies obtained from patients either at operation or by the percutaneous needle technique in Birmingham (Eade *et al.*, 1971) and in Oxford (Perrett *et al.*, 1971). Caution must be exercised in assessing the results of these more recent investigations. Each series included patients with disease in different parts of the intestinal tract. Two-thirds of the Birmingham series attended as out-patients for their hepatic studies, which suggests that they were not seriously ill from Crohn's disease at the time. More than

70 per cent of the Oxford patients had had earlier operations; one-third already had had a resection. Changes observed in a distant organ can be the result of treatment, as well as of the primary disease. Biochemical abnormality only becomes apparent when the very considerable reserve of hepatic function has been exhausted. Finally, there is considerable doubt as to how representative any one hepatic needle biopsy specimen may be. It is known that in the colon a great many sections must sometimes be cut and examined before an epithelioid-cell granuloma is seen. Failure to demonstrate granulomas on a liver biopsy does not mean that that organ is normal—the needle may simply have missed the affected part.

Approximately 25 per cent of the Birmingham and Oxford patients had biochemical evidence of liver dysfunction. No patient had a raised serum bilirubin (above 1·1 mg per 100 ml) at the time they were specially studied (Eade *et al.*, 1971), although 14 per cent stated that they had had jaundice in the past (Perrett *et al.*, 1971). Nine out of the 175 Aberdeen patients gave a history of previous jaundice. Serum alkaline phosphatase exceeded 15 King–Armstrong units in 14 per cent of the English patients, but appeared to be coming from bone rather than liver. Some of those with high levels had evidence of osteomalacia. The 5-nucleo-tidase concentration, a more specific index of hepatic cell function, was normal in 10 out of the 14 patients with raised serum alkaline phosphatase. Both groups of workers found the transaminase estimations unhelpful, and there was little or no correlation between biochemical disturbance and the histological state of the liver. When Crohn's disease had been present for more than 10 years, there was more likely to be retention of bromsulphthalein (BSP). Some degree of BSP retention was noted in 25 per cent. The disease was of long duration when more than 10 per cent was retained at 45 minutes, in 8 out of 9 cases. Age at onset, sex, ingestion of alcohol or drugs, immune reactions, and previous blood transfusions appeared to have no effect in determining whether the function of the liver and its microscopical appearance were normal or not.

The Oxford and Birmingham workers disagree on their histological findings. The former state that pathological changes were detected in only 50 per cent, whereas nearly all the Birmingham patients showed some abnormality. Small intestine disease damages the liver less than does its colonic counterpart. Infiltration with inflammatory cells, mainly lymphocytes, and fibrosis were seen in 71 per cent of all liver biopsy specimens (Eade *et al.*, 1971). The infiltrate was around and in the vicinity of the distributaries of the portal vein. It was related to the severity of the intestinal disease. The fibrous tissue rarely arranged itself concentrically, as in pericholangitis. However, Perrett *et al.* (1971) found 20 per cent of the Oxford patients on whom liver biopsies were performed had pericholangitis. Fibrosis is associated with bile duct proliferation. Kupffer cells are often prominent. Eight to 15 per cent of patients have focal cell necrosis. However, cirrhosis is rare; only 2–3 per cent of patients with Crohn's disease have it. When there is clinically overt liver disease, serum biochemical derangements are the rule.

Fatty infiltration is common, being seen in up to 40 per cent of cases; this observation had been made by earlier investigators (Rappaport *et al.*, 1951; Chapin *et al.*, 1956; Bacon and Pezzutti, 1966). Deposition of amyloid within the liver is a very uncommon feature, present in only about 2 per cent of living patients. In an autopsy series Werther *et al.* (1960) detected amyloid in 29 per cent, but this high incidence was almost certainly accounted for by the very severe and prolonged disease, with multiple operations and recurrent sepsis, which had finally killed their patients. Quite apart from the liver, when tnere is long-standing Crohn's disease, amyloidosis may in rare instances be widespread in the body and involve the kidneys, giving rise to a nephrotic syndrome and terminal uraemia (Brownstein, 1968).

Granulomas close to the portal tracts are seen in some patients. Dordal and colleagues (1967) in Chicago were able to demonstrate them in over 20 per cent of cases, but in Birmingham they were less common, 6 per cent of biopsy specimens showing them. Granulomas may disappear after a successful intestinal resection. However, their apparent resolution may be accounted for by the biopsy needle's sampling error.

Cultures of excised liver tissue and of portal venous blood (Eade *et al.*, 1971b) have given negative results, the few organisms grown almost certainly being contaminants (Perrett *et al.*, 1971). In contradistinction almost one-quarter of patients with ulcerative colitis are said to have positive portal blood cultures; adequate controls are necessary. The liver changes in patients with colonic Crohn's disease, particularly in those with the entire colon involved, are essentially similar to the changes met with in the mucosal form of colitis. There may be bridging hepato-fibrosis and sometimes granulomas. No satisfactory explanation for the failure to find bacteria in portal blood in Crohn's disease has been produced. Ulcerative colitis is essentially a mucosal disease, with widespread ulceration giving relatively easy access for luminal micro-organisms to small veins in the colon wall. The denuded surface area is probably much smaller in Crohn's disease, and the wall considerably thicker; the mucosa may remain intact while, away from the lumen, a non-bacterial type of inflammatory response is taking place in the submucosa. It may be a product of inflammation rather than pathogenic bacteria, which damages the liver. Excision of the inflamed bowel permits healing to take place (Maurer *et al.*, 1967).

One patient in the Aberdeen series developed a liver abscess; it was discovered at autopsy, along with several small intra-peritoneal and lung abscesses. According to Eade *et al.* (1971a) no liver abscess was found in 275 Birmingham patients. With the availability of broad-spectrum antibiotics, portal pyaemia and intra-hepatic abscess must now be very rare. Two liver abscesses were reported from Chicago (Sparberg *et al.*, 1966) in patients with Crohn's disease. Rigors, hectic pyrexia and drenching sweats are characteristic of a liver abscess. Jaundice is not a necessary part of the clinical picture. A hepatic scan and arteriography are helpful in making the diagnosis. The Mount Sinai Hospital doctors (Lerman *et al.*, 1962) described a case of pyelo-phlebitis progressing to abscess formation, the only example encountered in the very large number of patients with Crohn's disease who have attended that famous New York hospital. Earlier, Taylor (1949) had recounted a similar grim sequence of events.

Despite the recent upsurge of interest in them, hepatic changes still have little influence on the management of patients with Crohn's disease, at least in the early stages.

Cholelithiasis
The entero-hepatic circulation of bile salts depends on an intact terminal ileum where normally the bile salts that have been secreted by the liver are reabsorbed. Normally less than 1 gm of bile salts reaches the large intestine in 24 hours—the recycling system is almost closed. In Crohn's disease this quantity may be considerably exceeded even though intestinal transit time remains normal. Surgical removal of the distal ileum likewise increases the amount of bile salts escaping from the entero-hepatic circulation and, in addition, transit is expedited (Meihoff and Kern, 1968). There is a wide spectrum of change in bile salt meta-bolism—from severe impairment to near normality (Garbutt *et al.*, 1970). Probably some compensatory mechanisms slowly develop but they are not fully understood. In general there is only a small reduction in the total bile salt pool (Abaurre *et al.*, 1969).

When bile salts are being lost through the large bowel, their synthesis by the liver is increased (Hofmann, 1967). Nevertheless, their concentration in newly formed bile will probably decrease. As a result other solutes in the bile may precipitate out of the supersaturated solution, forming gallstones. The natural history of untreated Crohn's disease has to date provided little evidence to substantiate this theory. In an autopsy series Chapin *et al.* (1956) at the Mayo Clinic found gallstones in 12·8 per cent of patients dying with Crohn's disease, an incidence almost identical to that recorded in a normal population in Bristol, England (Heaton and Read, 1969). The American patients had had severe intestinal lesions and many had had operations. If and when satisfactory non-operative methods of controlling Crohn's disease are discovered, it will be possible to determine the incidence of gallstones after 5–10 years in patients who have retained their damaged ileum.

At present it would appear that removal of, or short-circuiting, the terminal ileum has more effect on gallstone formation than does granulomatous disease. Heaton and Read (1968) performed cholecysto-grams on 72 patients who had had from 30–120 cm of ileum resected or bypassed at least 18 months previously. Including patients who already had had cholecystectomies, the overall incidence of gallstones was 31·9 per cent, rising to 75 per cent in those who were followed up for more than 15 years. As in the general population, females were affected twice as often as males. Gallstones are usually non-opaque and more com-mon in the elderly, but after ileal surgery age did not affect the incidence and slightly more than half the stones were radio-opaque. Bile aspirated from the duodenum of a normal subject has a glycine to taurine con-jugation ratio varying between 2:1 to 6:1; in patients operated upon for Crohn's disease and who later formed stones, the ratio rose to a mean value of 12:1, possibly due to a lack of available taurine.

Cohen *et al.* (1971) have also recorded a high incidence of gallstones, 34 per cent, in patients who had had treatment for Crohn's disease 10 years earlier. Cholecystograms were performed in 28 Aberdeen patients 1–5 years after resection; only 2 patients had stones, which were causing no trouble and the gallbladders retained some function. Clearly a long time interval must elapse between operation and the formation of biliary calculi.

Removal of the normal site of absorption permits bile salts to enter the colon, where they have a cathartic effect, interfere with water absorption and so increase the water content of the stools (Hofmann, 1967). With stasis in a blind loop after bypass surgery and in the colon excessive bacterial degradation of bile salts may occur. Heaton and Read (1969) have suggested that a degradation product, lithocholic acid, may be responsible for gallstone formation. When there is a high glycine to taurine ratio it tends to form calcium salts which would be capable of producing radio-opaque stones.

Fortunately for the patients many of the gallstones detected very many years after operations for Crohn's disease are symptomless. Cholecystectomy is not indicated unless new symptoms are unquestion-ably arising from the gallbladder.

Ophthalmic Complications

Gastroenterologists and surgeons dealing with inflammatory bowel disease are well acquainted with the red eye and other ocular mani-festations of Crohn's disease. The expert opinion of an ophthalmologist is not usually sought. As a result no detailed study of the eye compli-cations has been made. Macoul (1970), in describing a boy with granulomatous ileocolitis who had recurrent conjunctivitis, irido-cyclitis and severe neuroretinitis, mentioned corneal ulcers, keratitis, episcleritis and lid oedema as being other complications sometimes present in Crohn's disease. Corlitz and Colls (1967) considered uveitis (iritis) in both ulcerative and transmural colitis. These two reports appear to be the only ones specifically on ocular changes. Twelve Aberdeen patients (7 per cent) were noted by their physician or surgeon to have eye lesions, which often lasted only a few days and did not require expert attention. Five were regarded as having episcleritis; corneal ulcers, keratitis, recurrent conjunctivitis and iridocyclitis were each diagnosed in one patient. Both cornea and sclera appeared to be involved in 2 cases, while insufficient information had been recorded about the twelfth patient to enable any retrospective diagnosis to be made. Six out of the 12 patients had arthritis or spondylitis. It is almost certain that careful questioning and expert examination of the eyes of patients with Crohn's disease would reveal a higher incidence of ocular complications. With slit lamp examination 19 per cent of the Oxford series were cosidered to have iritis (Perrett *et al.*, 1971).

Orthopaedic Complications

Arthritis. Among the 600 patients at the Mayo Clinic there was a 4·5 per cent incidence of arthritis (Van Patter *et al.*, 1954). In the West London areas, Ansell and Wigley (1964) studied 91 patients with Crohn's disease. Six patients had arthritis active at the time of the survey, but on detailed questioning about earlier joint symptoms, in all 33 patients apparently had had arthritis.

The joints affected, in asymmetrical fashion, are commonly the knee, ankle or wrist (Soren, 1966). Swelling and pain are the main features, and the arthritis tends to migrate from one large joint to another in the course of a few weeks. Bowel symptoms precede the development of painful joints, but once established the course of the polyarthritis frequently parallels the activity of the intestinal disease. The serum uric acid level is normal and the rheumatoid arthritis latex test is negative. Biopsy of the joint lining may show chronic inflammatory cell infiltrate, loss of synovial cell lining in places and some fibrinoid necrosis. How, ever, it is remarkable that there is no permanent damage to the joint once the attack has passed. There may be associated skin and eye lesions, for example erythema nodosum and uveitis.

Twenty-three of the Aberdeen clinical series of 175 patients had orthopaedic complaints (excluding the 5 cases of psoas abscess). Migratory polyarthritis was seen in 12 of these patients, an incidence of 6·8 per cent which is very similar to that observed by Ansell and Wigley (1964). Crohn's disease came first in all cases. It was unusual for a joint to look red for more than a few days, but the effusion some-times lasted for several weeks. Three of the 12 patients had erythema nodosum and one had eczema. Five had either episcleritis or uveitis (iritis).

Intensive medical therapy, including steroids, produced an ameliora-
tion of joint (and bowel) symptoms in most instances. Nevertheless,
attacks recurred until all diseased intestinal tissue had been excised.

Spondylitis and Sacro-iliitis. Acheson (1960), from a review of discharges of male patients from the U.S. Veterans' Administration
hospitals, concluded that 3 per cent of those diagnosed as suffering
from Crohn's disease also had spondylitis. This was a much higher
incidence than could be accounted for by chance. Ansell and Wigley
(1964) believed that up to 6 per cent of their patients had spondylitis.
The incidence of erosion and sclerosis at the sacro-iliac joints may be 2
or 3 times that of the spinal abnormality; in the Oxford series it reached
15 per cent (Perrett *et al.*, 1971). Special films of the joints are desirable.
More than half the patients have had back pain for a long time before
intestinal disease becomes apparent. Radiological changes may be
discernible in the small intestine when the patient's bowel is still
functioning normally (McBride *et al.*, 1963).

The usual complaint is of low back pain and morning stiffness made
worse by exertion, especially bending. There may be tenderness over one
or both sacro-iliac joints. Unlike full-blown ankylosing spondylitis, in
inflammatory bowel disease the spondylitis has little tendency to spread
up the spine and the costo-vertebral articulations are not affected—
chest expansion is mostly normal. However, a familial factor may be
involved in the aetiology of both conditions, first degree relatives
showing an increased incidence of bowel or spinal disease (McBride *et
al.*, 1963). Patients with Crohn's disease who have spondylitis may in
addition have migratory arthritis or uveal tract inflammation (Acheson,
1960).

Six of the Aberdeen clinical series of 175 patints were believed to
have spondylitis, an incidence of 3·4 per cent. Four other patients did
complain of low back pain, but no definite diagnosis was made. Routine
X-rays of sacro-iliac joints have not been carried out, so that it is not
known how frequently they were involved. Of the 6 patients with
spondylitis, 3 were men and 3 were women—when they have inflammatory bowel disease females seem to suffer relatively more frequently
from spondylitis than they do when otherwise healthy. Three of the
patients received treatment for their back complaints more than 12
years ago and old X-ray films are no longer available. However, 2 of the
3 were given a course of radiotherapy, so it is reasonable to assume that
the diagnosis had been carefully made. Four of the patients had been
troubled with their backs for up to 7 years before noticing any bowel
disturbance. The mother of one of these patients had had a resection
for Crohn's disease about 20 years earlier, the only example of the
familial occurrence of the disease in the Aberdeen series. One patient
first felt pain and stiffness in his back some months after starting medical

treatment for his granulomatous enteritis. Crohn's disease was found
in the sixth patient when barium studies were performed to ascertain if
there was any intestinal cause for his spondylitis (Fig. 2). In one 24-
year-old female the disease was further complicated by episcleritis and
an eczematous rash.

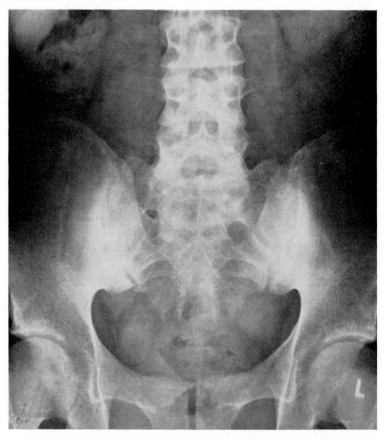

FIG. 2. Sacro-iliitis. Sclerosis of the bone and partial obliteration of the
sacro-iliac joints in a patient who, when being investigated for low back
pain, was found to have Crohn's disease.

Radiotherapy did help the 2 patients who received it; they were
having very little trouble with their backs while attending hospital
years afterwards with Crohn's disease. Medical treatment of the
intestinal lesion was not very effective in relieving co-existing back
symptoms unless large doses of corticosteroids were administered.

Other Bone and Joint Lesions. Osteomyelitis of the ilium and of the fifth lumbar vertebra, associated with large abscesses, was treated in Chicago by Goldstein *et al.* (1969). A pelvic abscess in Crohn's disease may also spread to the hip joint, giving rise to septic arthritis (London and Fitton, 1970); amputation through the hip may be necessary in order to save life. Retardation of growth is to be expected in children with Crohn's disease. However, Neale *et al.* (1968) had a boy of 17 years who had developed severe Crohn's disease five years earlier. During that time his height had increased by 27 cm to 185 cm. Laminated periosteal new bone formation was seen on X-rays of the long bones of his legs and forearms. The incidence and cause of this type of diffuse periostitis are not known.

Necrosis of the femoral head thought to be due to Crohn's disease rather than to its treatment by steroids has been reported (Brom *et al.*, 1971). One Aberdeen girl, who did not have particularly severe Crohn's disease, was found to have marked generalized osteoporosis. Her condition improved rapidly after ileal resection and she has remained well for 7 years.

Urological Complications

Fistulae. Ileo-vesical fistulae in Crohn's disease are discussed on page 127. It is possible to get complex fistulae from sigmoid colon into the bladder (Mellin, 1959); recently a uretero-ileal fistula has been described in a 25-year-old male who had suffered from Crohn's disease for 2 years (Blumgart and Thakur, 1971). None of these fistulae is common. It is probable that persistent or recurrent urinary infections occur more frequently, but no accurate figures regarding their incidence are available. In a proportion of patients with Crohn's disease the inflamed ileum must lie in contact with the dome or lateral wall of the bladder; a small juxtavesical abscess may develop. If untreated, the inflammatory process may form a fistula.

Stones. Nephrolithiasis and obstructive uropathy are more common complications of Crohn's disease than fistulae into the urinary tract. There is a difference of opinion regarding their respective frequencies of occurrence. At the Lahey Clinic, with ileal disease the incidence of renal calculi was 3·6 per cent, rising to 10·3 per cent when the colon was involved (Vantrappen *et al.*, 1966). Seven per cent of the Belgian patients at Louvain who had Crohn's ileo-colitis developed renal calculi. In J. B. Kirsner's clinic in Chicago, stones were present in 10·9 per cent of those with small intestinal disease, compared to 9·3 per cent of patients with transmural colitis and only 6·4 per cent in a series of 677 ulcerative colitics. Most of the ileal Crohn's disease patients were males, the average duration of symptoms being 11·6 years (Gelzayd *et al.*, 1968). At the Mount Sinai Hospital, New York, there were 28 cases of nephrolithiasis in a total of 583 patients with inflammatory bowel disease (4·8 per cent). It is interesting that when an ileostomy is established after a colectomy, the stone incidence rises as high as 13 per cent (Maratka and Nedbal, 1964). Five out of 17 patients with uric acid stones studied by Badenoch (1960) had had ulcerative colitis, and 4 of them had had ileostomies. Two Aberdeen patients had operations for triple phosphate stones, one before and one after commencing treatment for Crohn's disease. Another female developed an oxalate stone 2 years after a short-circuit with exclusion had been performed. The stone was removed from the left renal pelvis, but she continues to have symptoms from her Crohn's disease.

Several factors may be involved in the aetiology of renal calculi in Crohn's disease. Breuer *et al.* (1970) have shown that the 24 hour output and concentration of both uric acid and calcium in the urine are increased in granulomatous disease of the intestine. Recumbency and steroid therapy also increase calcium output. Stasis from ureteric obstruction (*vide infra*) possibly plays a role when stones form in the right kidney; upper urinary tract infection does not seem to be as important as might be expected. Hofmann *et al.* (1970) have suggested that the excess oxalate that they detected in the urine of 2 patients may have been derived from the glycine moiety of the somewhat increased amount of glycine-conjugated bile salts present after ileal resection.

Hydronephrosis. Obstruction of the middle portion of the ureter by retroperitoneal spread of inflammation in Crohn's disease has been well documented in recent years (Schofield *et al.*, 1968; Present *et al.*, 1969; Enker and Block, 1970). Although Hyams *et al.* gave the first description of it in 1943, this complication has not always been recognized. Two Aberdeen patients had nephrectomies for gross right-sided hydronephrosis before it was appreciated that ileal inflammation was responsible. Recurrent Crohn's disease after a right hemi-colectomy obstructed the ureter of a third patient.

Ten patients with obstructive hydronephrosis were detected among 150 New York patients (6·6 per cent) studied by Present and his colleagues. They remarked on how few symptoms and how little laboratory evidence there was of urinary tract infection. Pain in the groin and front of the right thigh from nerve irritation was more troublesome. In Manchester, Schofield found only 2 examples of ureteral involvement among 188 patients. However, when radio-active renography (Hippuran-I[131]) was performed on 10 patients free from urinary symptoms, there was some evidence of ureteral stasis on the right side in 5, and 2 of these also had some hold-up in the proximal part of the left ureter.

Enker and Block (1970) likened the peri-ureteric fibrosis to pseudo-myxomatous tissue. They have performed formal ureterolysis and ileal resection successfully in 6 patients. The thickened area of retroperitoneal tissue is incised longitudinally—and if need be a wedge is excised—so as to leave the ureter bare on its anterior aspect, without any likelihood of the fibrous process constricting it once again. Results of this more radical operation have been better than those achieved by ileal short-circuit plus exclusion. The dilatation of the upper urinary tract starts to diminish in 7–10 days.

Perforation

More than 100 free perforations into the peritoneal cavity have now been recorded. In 1968 Kyle *et al.* were able to collect information about 91 cases, and described 4 more seen in Aberdeen. Two further

Table 3

Free perforation complicating Crohn's disease in north-east Scotland

No.	Sex	Age	Site	Therapy	Result
1	F	60	Lower ileum	Resection	Recurred after 7 years
2	M	24	Mid ileum	Suture	Well. External fistula
3	F	22	Terminal ileum	Suture	Resected 1 year later
4	F	26	Proximal and mid ileum	—	Sudden death
5	F	38	Terminal ileum	Resection	Well
6	F	45	Terminal ileum	Resection	Died

perforations have been recognized, making a total of 6 among approximately 200 patients with Crohn's disease treated in north-east Scotland up to the end of 1971. This incidence of 3 per cent is becoming standard in large series of cases with Crohn's disease (Edwards, 1964; Colcock, 1965). Details of the Scottish patients are given in Table 3. Perforation can take place in any age and at any stage of the disease. Four out of the 6 Aberdeen patients were known to have chronic granulomatous disease of the intestine. The first and last cases perforated unexpectedly, although there was a history of earlier diarrhoea. Crohn (1965) has described several perforations in acute regional enteritis. Two Scottish patients perforated while in hospital; Case 4 was gravely ill with a condition comparable to enteritis gravis (Buckley *et al.*, 1962; Mogadam and Priest, 1969) when she collapsed and died before laparotomy could be performed. None of the patients had had steroids within the preceding 3 months.

The perforations that have been described have almost all been in the small intestine. Waye and Lithgow (1967) have had a perforation in an excluded loop of ileum after bypass surgery. Acute perforation of the colon in Crohn's disease is rare (Babb *et al.*, 1970), but reports are beginning to appear (Javett and Brooke, 1971; Shahmanesh and Wilken, 1971) and are likely to increase with more general recognition of colonic forms of the disease. The opening in jejunum or ileum may be on the mesenteric side or, less frequently, on the anti-mesenteric border of the thickened bowel. In Case 2 perforation had taken place in un-healthy, dilated ileum proximal to a stenosed segment. Two of the Aberdeen patients had perforated simultaneously in two places. Urca (1971) reported a 56 year old male said to have perforated twice, but on the second occasion the perforation seems to have been localized, with abscess formation.

The exact mechanism of perforation is not known. A large fissure may slowly erode its way through the grossly thickened wall, the visceral peritoneum then giving way suddenly. With acute types of enteritis an ulcer may rapidly erode the wall. Another explanation is that there is a small infarct of part of the intestinal wall (Harjola *et al.*, 1965); the area of necrosis finally ruptures and generalized peritonitis follows. Obstruction may sometimes play a part.

The clinical features are similar to those of free perforation of an anterior duodenal ulcer. There is acute abdominal pain, with tenderness and marked muscular guarding, particularly in the lower abdomen. An X-ray taken with the patient in the erect position may show gas under the diaphragm; this finding is not so constant as it is with duodenal or gastric perforation. Vigorous resuscitation is necessary. Drainage, simple suture, short-circuiting and emergency resection have all been employed in the treatment of perforated Crohn's disease; when feasible an adequate resection is probably the best treatment. Case 7 had been receiving medical treatment for 2 years, and died following an emer-gency resection. Her life might well have been saved if elective removal of her localized lesion had been carried out at an earlier stage in her disease.

Haemorrhage

Crohn and Yarnis (1958) listed 25 patients out of a series of 526 as having experienced gross rectal bleeding. Fourteen out of the 600 patients at the Mayo Clinic had profuse red blood in their stools (Van Patter *et al.*, 1954). Other sources of haemorrhage in the gastro-intestinal tract were not always excluded: some of the New York patients could have been bleeding from the peptic ulcers that they were known to have. In Chicago, Sparberg and Kirsner (1966) from a series of 195 patients, had 7 patients who bled. They described 3 of these patients who each had 5 or more haemorrhages. Lesions of the small intestine are rare causes of gastrointestinal bleeding. Even when the source is in the small bowel, Crohn's disease accounts for less than 4 per cent of the total (Netterville *et al.*, 1968). More bleeding might be anticipated with disease of the colon, and while it occurs (Goldberg and Frahle, 1963) it is much less common than in ulcerative colitis.

Only one Aberdeen patient presented at the Out Patient Clinic on account of rectal bleeding some days previously. No other patient has had a major haemorrhage. Considering the extent of the mucosal ulceration, the very prolonged course of the disease, and the large oedematous haemorrhoids produced by persistent diarrhoea, more rectal bleeding might have been anticipated. Slow continuous blood loss is much more of a problem than catastrophic haemorrhage.

It is always difficult to define massive, life-threatening gastrointestinal haemorrhage. The patient should be in a state of clinical shock, with a systolic blood pressure under 100 mm Hg and a haemoglobin of less than 9 gm per 100 ml. Sauter, in 1966, stated that only 18 patients suffering massive haemorrhage from Crohn's disease has been reported. No details were available about several patients, and others probably did not meet all the criteria given above.

In the unlikely event of being confronted with a patient suffering a massive haemorrhage, it would be advisable to transfuse him rapidly, controlling the rate by CVP measurements, until his blood pressure is normal. Corticosteroids may be given. When hypovolaemia has been corrected, the patient is observed: if he requires more than 500 ml of transfused blood in a 4-hour period to keep his vital parameters normal, then resection should be undertaken without further loss of time.

Toxic Megacolon

Writing in 1966, Janowitz and his colleagues from Mount Sinai Hospital stated that toxic dilatation of the colon, well known as a grave complication of ulcerative colitis, did not occur in transmural colitis. A year later, Korelitz, from the same hospital, when describing the clinical course "of inflammatory disease initially sparing the rectum" mentioned 3 cases with toxic megacolon out of a total series of 94 patients. In their classical paper on the differentiation between Crohn's disease and proctocolitis, Lennard-Jones *et al.* (1971) stated that toxic megacolon could appear in the former type of colitis, but some workers still regard it as rare (Zetzel, 1971). The highest incidence of toxic megacolon has been recorded at the Cleveland Clinic where Hawk and Turnbull (1966) stated that 16 per cent had the complication. No details were given, but later Farmer *et al.* (1967) stated that granulomas were found in 4 out of the 14 patients. The Cleveland Clinic has re-classified as Crohn's disease many colons originally resected in the belief that they were ulcerative colitis.

Schacter *et al.* (1967) were the first to give a comprehensive account of megacolon in a patient with Crohn's disease and there was another example in the series reported by McGovern and Goulston (1968). The largest number of cases described in detail were from St George's Hospital, London. There Javett and Brooke (1970) dealt with 5 patients with acute dilatation of the colon, one of whom had 2 free perforations. Their ages ranged from 20 to 64 years, all had had symptoms for months or years before toxic megacolon appeared, and the diagnosis of Crohn's disease was confirmed in all cases. The patients were very ill, with fever, tachycardia and toxaemia. Four had emergency colectomies, with removal of the rectal stump some time later. All 5 survived. Papp and Pollard (1971) from Ann Arbor, have had a 19-year-old male and a 19-year-old female with toxic megacolon. The female had 2 attacks of acute dilatation more than 26 months apart.

A 25-year-old female presented in Aberdeen in June, 1971, with a 6 months' history of diarrhoea and weight loss. Upper abdominal pain and erythema nodosum had appeared during the 6 weeks prior to admission to hospital. The patient was drowsy and confused, running a high fever and with a tympanitic upper abdomen. Straight X-ray showed the transverse colon to be 5 cm in diameter. A few punctate and small linear ulcers were seen on sigmoidoscopy. Biopsy of one of these showed oedema and lymphoid aggregates in the submucosa and early granulomatous change. The patient responded slowly to intravenous fluids, blood transfusion, corticosteroids and cephaloridine. When she had improved, a barium meal and follow-through showed marked inflammatory changes both in the small and in the large intestine.

The thickening and fibrosis which are characteristic of transmural colitis apparently are unable to prevent dilatation even when they are of long standing. There is no evidence that antispasmodic drugs, steroids or the performance of a barium enema precipitate an attack of toxic megacolon. The exact cause and mechanism of dilatation remain unknown. The most energetic treatment is required if the patient's life is to be saved.

Cancer

Carcinoma complicating Crohn's disease both in the ileum (Shiel *et al.*, 1968; Tyers *et al.*, 1969) and in the colon (Perrett *et al.*, 1968; Jones, 1969) is now well documented. Rha *et al.* (1971) collected reports of 20 ileal carcinomas from the literature. In nearly all cases, Crohn's disease had been of long standing, the mean duration being 14·3 years. In the general population, malignant tumours of the small intestine are rare; many are sarcomatous and situated in the jejunum (McPeak, 1967). When the patient has had Crohn's disease the tumour is an adeno-carcinoma, mostly in the terminal ileum, and on average patients are 12 years younger than ordinary patients with small intestinal carcinomas. Rha *et al.* (1971) at laparotomy did not realize that the red, thickened ileum of their own patient contained a carcinoma; it was discovered on histological examination. Therefore it seems likely that in the past some tumours may have been overlooked. Brown *et al.* (1970) described the sixth case where an adenocarcinoma had arisen in ileum many years after bypass surgery. Even exclusion of the ileum does not protect it from the danger of cancer (Schuman, 1970), and because of the lingering risk, Bloquiaux (1968) recommended resection instead of short-circuiting procedures in the treatment of Crohn's disease.

Shiel *et al.* (1968) investigated the possible relationship between the chronic intestinal inflammation and the appearance of a carcinoma. The long antecedent history of Crohn's disease, the early age at onset and the location of the tumours suggested that the association was closer than could be accounted for by chance. Patients with isolated and uncomplicated small intestinal carcinomas had none of the microscopic changes of Crohn's disease in the tissues surrounding their tumours. There is a possibility that bacteria in areas of stasis may alter bile salts and produce a carcinogen.

Reticulum-cell sarcoma has been found in intestine affected by Crohn's disease (Hughes, 1955). Benign carcinoid tumours are occasionally noted in resected specimens of diseased ileum. Wood *et al.* (1970) presented what they believed to be the first description of co-existent Crohn's disease and malignant carcinoid tumour, with metastases in regional nodes. The latter type of tumour can closely simulate Crohn's disease both in its symptomatology and macroscopic appearance (Crohn and Yarnis, 1958).

Carcinoma of the colon is a very common disease, and by chance a patient who had had Crohn's disease in the terminal ileum might later develop a neoplasm in colon or rectum (Davis and Caley, 1960). It is much more difficult to evaluate the relationship when a carcinoma is found in a colon (or rectum) affected by Crohn's disease. In one of the Aberdeen patients there was a small rectal carcinoma at the lower border of a segment showing the classical histological changes of transmural colitis. Jones (1969) described 4 patients from St Mark's Hospital, London, who had both Crohn's disease and carcinoma of colon. He concluded that the available evidence did not establish an increased risk of malignancy in colonic Crohn's disease. However, few patients have been followed up for over 10 years and as Jones pointed out, in 90 per cent the diseased colon has been excised within that time. At Oxford there were 3 cases of carcinoma in 82 patients with colonic involvement by Crohn's disease (Perrett *et al.*, 1968), an incidence of 3·7 per cent. This figure corresponds closely with the 3·5 per cent incidence of carcinoma recorded at the same hospital in patients with ulcerative colitis. The risk of carcinoma developing after many years in ulcerative colitis is well known. Patients with Crohn's disease of the colon who do not have resections will require careful supervision in case cancer finally supervenes.

Bile duct carcinoma has been described in patients with ulcerative colitis and may be related to long-standing pericholangitis (Converse *et al.*, 1971). No report of such a neoplasm in colonic Crohn's disease has been seen up to the end of 1971.

References

Abaurre, R., Gordon, S. G., Mann, J. G. and Kern, F. (1969), *Gastroenterology*, **57** 679.
Acheson, E. D. (1960), *Quart. J. Med.*, **29**, 489.
Ansell, B. M. and Wigley, R. A. D. (1964), *Ann. Rheum. Dis.*, **23**, 64.
Atwell, J. D., Duthie, H. L. and Goligher, J. C. (1965), *Brit. J. Surg.*, **52**, 966.
Babb, R. R., Kieraldo, J. H. and Vescia, F. G. (1970), *Amer. J. Dig. Dis.*, **15**, 573.
Bacon, H. E. and Pezzutti, J. E. (1966), *J. Amer. med. Ass.*, **198**, 1330.
Badenoch, A. W. (1960), *Brit. J. Urol.*, **32**, 374.
Bloquiaux, W. (1968), *Tijd. v. Gastro-Ent.*, **11**, 496.
Blumgart, L. H. and Thakur, K. (1971), *Brit. J. Surg.*, **58**, 469.
Bowen, G. H. and Kirsner, J. B. (1965), *Med. Clin. N. Amer.*, **49**, 17.
Breuer, R. I., Gelzayd, E. A. and Kirsner, J. B. (1970), *Gut*, **11**, 319.
Brom, B., Bank, S., Marks, I. N. and Cobb, J. J. (1971), *Gastroenterology*, **60**, 1106.
Brown, N., Weinstein, V. A. and Janowitz, H. D. (1970), *Mt. Sinai J. Med.*, **37**, 675.
Brownstein, M. H. (1968), *J. New York J. Med.*, **68**, 1069.
Buckley, J. J., Sieden, S. P., Jiminez, F. A. and Kaufman, G.(1962), *Gastroenterology*, **42**, 330.
Chapin, L. E., Scudamore, H. H., Bagenstosse, A. H. and Bargen, J. A. (1956), *Gastroenterology*, **30**, 404.
Cohen, S., Kaplan, M., Gottlieb, L. and Patterson, J. (1971), *Gastroenterology*, **60**, 237.
Colcock, B. P. (1965), "Regional Enteritis". *Current Problems in Surgery*. Chicago, Year Book Medical Publishers.
Converse, C. F., Reagan, J. W. and DeCosse, J. J. (1971), *Amer. J. Surg.*, **121**, 39.
Corlitz, B. I. and Colls, R. S. (1967), *Gastroenterology*, **52**, 78.
Cornes, J. S. and Stecher, M. (1961), *Gut*, **2**, 189.
Cornet, A., Steg, A., Terris, G. and Laverdant, C. (1963), *Sem. Hop. Paris*, **29**, 1766.
Crohn, B. B. and Yarnis, H. (1958), *Regional Ileitis*, 2nd Edit. New York, Grune and Stratton.
Crohn, B. B. (1965), *New York J. Med.*, **65**, 641.
Davis, A. and Caley, J. P. (1960), *Postgrad. med. J.*, **36**, 380.
Davis, S. E. and Sperling, L. (1969), *Arch. Surg.*, **99**, 424.
de Dombal, F. T., Burton, I. and Goligher, J. C. (1971), *Brit. J. Surg.*, **58**, 805.
Dordal, E., Glagov, S. and Kirsner, J. B. (1967), *Gastroenterology*, **52**, 239.
Eade, M. N., Cooke, W. T. and Williams, J. A. (1971), *Scand. J. Gastroent.*, **6**, 199.
Eade, M. N., Cooke, W. T., Brooke, B. N. and Thompson, H. (1971b), *Ann. Int. Med.*, **74**, 518.
Edwards, H. (1964), *J. roy. Coll. Surg. Edin.*, **2**, 115.
Enker, W. E. and Block, G. E. (1970), *Arch. Surg. (Chicago)*, **101**, 319.
Garbutt, J. T., Wilkins, R. M., Lack, L. and Tyor, M. P. (1970), *Gastroenterology*, **59**, 551.
Gelzayd, E. A., Breuer, R. I. and Kirsner, J. B. (1968), *Amer. J. Dig. Dis.*, **13**, 1027.
Goldberg, S. L. and Frable, M. A. (1963), *Surgery*, **53**, 612.
Goldstein, M. J., Nasr, K., Singer, H. C., Anderson, J. G. D. and Kirsner, J. (1969), *Gut*, **10**, 264.
Grossman, M. S. and Nugent, F. W. (1967), *Amer. J. Dig. Dis.*, **12**, 491.
Harjola, P. T., Appelqvist, R. and Lilios, H. G. (1965), *Acta chir. Scand.*, **130**, 143.
Heaton, K. W. and Read, A. E. (1969), *Brit. med. J.*, **3**, 494.

Helms, C. H. and Bradshaw, H. H. (1964), *Surg. Gynec. Obstet.*, **119**, 330.
Hiley, P. C., Cohen, N. and Present, D. H. (1971), *Gastroenterology*, **60**, 103.
Hillman, R. S. and Henderson, P. A. (1969), *J. Clin. Investig.*, **48**, 453.
Hoffbrand, A. V., Tabaqchali, S., Booth, C. C. and Mollin, D. L. (1971), *Gut*, **12**, 27.
Hofmann, A. F. (1967), *Gastroenterology*, **52**, 752.
Hofmann, A. F., Thomas, P. J., Smith, L. H. and McCall, J. T. (1970), *Am. G.E. Ass. Boston*, **58**, 960.
Holzbach, R. T. (1969), *Amer. J. Gastroent.*, **52**, 48.
Hughes, R. K. (1955), *Amer. Surg.*, **21**, 770.
Hyams, J. A., Weinberg, S. A. and Alley, J. (1943), *Amer. J. Surg.*, **61**, 117.
Javett, S. L. and Brooke, B. N. (1971), *Lancet*, **2**, 126.
Jones, J. H. (1969), *Gut*, **10**, 651.
Kyle, J. (1971), *Gastroenterology*, **61**, 149.
Kyle, J., Caridis, T., Duncan, T. and Ewen, S. W. (1968), *Amer. J. Dig. Dis.*, **13**, 275.
Kyle, J. and Sinclair, W. Y. (1969), *Brit. J. Surg.*, **56**, 474.
Kyle, J. and Murray, C. M. (1969), *Surgery*, **66**, 497.
Lerman, B., Garlock, J. and Janowitz, H. (1962), *Ann. Surg.*, **155**, 441.
London, D. and Fitton, J. M. (1970), *Brit. J. Surg.*, **57**, 536.
Lorenzo, G. A. and Beal, J. M. (1969), *Arch. Surg.*, **99**, 394.
McBride, J., King, M., Baikie, A., Crean, G. and Sircus, W. (1963), *Brit. med. J.*, **2**, 483.
McPeak, C. J. (1967), *Amer. J. Surg.*, **114**, 402.
Macoul, K. L. (1970), *Arch. Ophthal. (Chicago)*, **84**, 95.
Mathews, J. E., Peterson, R. F., Eberts, J. P. and White, R. R. (1971), *Ann. Surg.*, **173**, 966.
Mazier, W. P. (1971), *Dis. Colon Rectum*, **14**, 134.
Meihoff, W. E. and Kern, F. (1968), *J. Clin. Investig.*, **47**, 261.
Melich, E. I. (1969), *Am. J. Gastroent.*, **52**, 231.
Mellin, P. (1959), *Med. Klin.*, **54**, 1456.
Mogadam, M. and Priest, R. J. (1969), *Gastroenterology*, **56**, 337.
Neale, G., Kelsall, A. R. and Doyle, F. H. (1968), *Gut*, **9**, 383.
Neely, J. C. (1962), *Amer. J. Surg.*, **103**, 119.
Netterville, R. E., Hardy, J. D., Martin, R. S. (1968), *Ann. Surg.*, **167**, 949.
Nygaard, K., Helsingen, N. and Rootwelt, K. (1970), *Scand. J. Gastroent.*, **5**, 349.
Pugh, H. L. (1945), *Ann. Surg.*, **122**, 845.
Perrett, A. D., Truelove, S. C. and Massarella, G. R. (1968), *Brit. med. J.*, **2**, 466.
Perrett, A. D., Higgins, G., Johnston, H. H., Massarella, G. R., Truelove, S. C. and Wright, R. (1971), *Quart. J. Med.*, **40**, 187.
Petersen, H., Myren, J. and Hertzberg, J. N. (1969), *Scand. J. Gastroent.*, **4**, 575.
Present, D. H., Rabinowitz, J. G., Banks P. A. and Janowitz, H. D. (1969), *New Engl. J. Med.*, **280**, 523.
Rampai, M., Briscot, R., Dor, V. and Guerinel, G. (1963), *Marseille Chir.*, **15**, 68.
Rappaport, H., Burgoyne, F. H. and Smetana, H. F. (1951), *Milit. Surg.*, **109**, 463.
Rha, C. K., Klein, N. C. and Wilson, J. M. (1971), *Arch. Surg. (Chicago)*, **102**, 630.
Richards, A. J., Condon, J. R. and Mallinson, C. N. (1971), *Brit. J. Surg.*, **58**, 493.
Sauter, K. E. (1966), *Amer. J. Surg.*, **112**, 91.
Scharf, V. (1969), *Ohio Med. J.*, **65**, 490.
Schofield, P. F. (1965), *Ann. roy. Coll. Surg. Engl.*, **36**, 258.
Schofield, P. F., Staff, W. G. and Moore, T. (1968), *J. Urol.*, **99**, 412.
Schuman, B. M. (1970), *New Engl. J. Med.*, **283**, 136.
Shahmanesh, M. and Wilken, B. J. (1970), *Lancet*, **2**, 363.
Sheil, F. O'M., Clark, C. G. and Goligher, J. C. (1968), *Brit. J. Surg.*, **55**, 53.
Sheldon, G. F., Gardiner, B. N., Way, L. W. and Dunphy, J. E. (1971), *Surg. Gynec. Obstet.*, **133**, 385.
Soren, A. (1966), *Arch. Int. Med. (Chicago)*, **117**, 78.

Sparberg, M. and Kirsner, J. B. (1966), *Amer. J. Dig. Dis.*, **11,** 652.

Taylor, F. W. (1949), *Amer. J. Med.*, **7,** 838.

Urca, I. (1971), *Dis. Colon Rectum*, **14,** 310.

Van Patter, W. N., Bargen, J. A., Dockerty, M. B., Feldman, W. H., Mayo, C. W. and Waugh, J. M. (1954), *Gastroenterology*, **26,** 347.

Waye, J. D. and Lithgow, C. (1967), *Gastroenterology*, **53,** 625.

Werther, J. L., Schapiro, A., Rubinstein, O. and Janowitz, H. D. (1960), *Amer. J. Med.*, **29,** 416.

Wood, W. J., Archer, R., Schaeffer, J. W., Stephens, C. and Griffen, W. (1970), *Gastroenterology*, **59,** 265.

Chapter VIII
Medical Treatment

The aim of treatment of a disease is to counteract and eliminate the cause and thereby to cure the patient. In Crohn's disease the cause is not known at present. Consequently the clinician's aims have to be modified and treatment is directed towards: (i) relieving symptoms; (ii) correcting deficiencies; and (iii) controlling or removing the more obvious pathological manifestations such as chronic inflammation in the bowel. These three lines of treatment are often pursued simultaneously; the third one includes surgery, discussed in Chapter IX. Removal of or short-circuit procedures on narrow, ulcerated intestine will greatly improve distressing symptoms and, unless excision has been carried to extremes, will prevent further deficiencies from developing. Unfortunately neither medical nor surgical treatment permanently cures Crohn's disease.

The variety and effectiveness of the drugs available to the physician have increased considerably during the past decade. Whereas formerly 90 per cent of patients with Crohn's disease were treated surgically, in 1972 at least 20 per cent of patients attending hospital are being treated by medical measures. Surgery may eventually be required, but it is now possible to keep patients comfortable for many months or years on drug treatment and nutritional supplements once the diagnosis has been established.

Unless they first present with acute obstruction or as acute appendicitis, most patients with Crohn's disease are initially treated by medical measures, and their progress is assessed at intervals. The other indications for prolonged medical management are: (a) when the onset has been insidious and the symptoms are mild, even though barium studies show definite abnormalities; (b) very widespread involvement of the bowel; (c) recurrence after adequate resection, except when it is causing obstruction; (d) other serious illness rendering the patient unfit for surgery.

One important aspect of Crohn's disease is its very chronic nature. Ideally the patient should probably be kept under some form of surveillance for the remainder of his life. The majority of patients are young adults—fathers trying to earn their living and mothers endeavouring to look after a family. Every effort must be made to enable these patients to lead as normal a life as possible. From time to time a critical look should be taken at the quality of life that each patient is leading, to see if medically it can be improved. These patients have the right to expect to be able to eat out in restaurants, to play games, have children, take holidays abroad, and to act like other people. Therapeutic advice must sometimes be tempered by the realities of the modern world.

Even after operation some of the advice given in the following section can usefully be followed. The course of the disease varies greatly. There are often relatively long periods when symptoms are minimal, but the patient is always liable to unpredictable exacerbations. Only general measures and maintenance therapy are required during a remission. When a relapse takes place medical therapy must be stepped up until the disease is once more under control.

General Measures

Activity
For most of the time men and women with Crohn's disease can proceed about their business. They can indulge in all normal forms of activity, but having an intestinal lesion, their nutrition may be suboptimal. It is important that they get adequate rest and sleep. Some patients are very conscientious and may take life too seriously. A good doctor should counsel them to relax a little and take things easier. Rest by itself on occasions seems to improve symptoms that are becoming troublesome. It is by no means certain whether it is bed rest or the passage of time alone that leads to symptomatic improvement. During a flare-up of their Crohn's disease, a few days' rest in bed is beneficial, possibly by lowering the demand for calories brought about by excessive catabolism. If the patient is having to stay off work and go to bed at frequent intervals, psychological problems may understandably arise. Fortunately this is rare, and with medical assistance most patients can continue to do a useful day's work.

Diet
By trial and error most patients gradually find out which foods agree with them and which aggravate diarrhoea or precipitate bouts of intestinal colic. Foodstuffs such as vegetables and fruit with a high residue content are liable to produce bolus colic. The brassica group of green vegetables and also peas and beans at one time had a bad reputation. However, some fresh fruit and vegetables, chewed thoroughly and eaten slowly, are desirable in any balanced diet; liquidized fruit preparations may be given. Without vitamin C the patient may become scorbutic.

With extensive disease, fat absorption is defective, and it may be advisable to restrict the fat intake in order to lessen steatorrhoea. Unfortunately this restriction would tend to deprive the patient of part of his richest source of calories. A very high carbohydrate diet often increases the frequency of bowel action. Irritant substances such as spices and alcoholic spirits also worsen diarrhoea in a proportion of patients, and are better avoided. Milk intolerance is unusual. There is no convincing evidence of a primary defect in handling lactose in Crohn's disease although a few patients may show it as a secondary phenomenon.

In general, patients who have any symptoms are better to keep to a high protein, low fat and low residue type of diet. It is difficult to achieve a very high protein intake; large quantities of protein tend to be nauseating and are certainly expensive. The patients' attempts to construct a suitable diet may lead to a deficient intake of calories and vitamins. The guidance of a dietitian is invaluable. A daily supply of 2,500 to 3,000 calories is required, depending on weight, activity, inflammation, etc. If eating food containing this number of calories at three main meals precipitates colic or diarrhoea, the patient is told to eat smaller amounts at more frequent intervals.

Relief of Symptoms

The two most common symptoms in Crohn's disease are colicky abdominal pain and diarrhoea. The dietary measures outlined above and treatment of the chronic inflammatory process will help control both symptoms. In addition, several more specific drugs are available for dealing with pain and diarrhoea.

Abdominal Pain

Codeine phosphate is a useful and safe drug, given orally in a dose of 15–45 mg. Not only does it relieve pain but it also reduces the tendency to diarrhoea. Pentazocine ("Fortral," Winthrop) is also used, the dose being 50 mg orally. If necessary, it can be administered intramuscularly. The regular use of a potent analgesic like pethidine is unwise. It is liable to mask the clinical findings of any complications, and it leads to addiction. Methadone ("Physeptone," Burroughs Wellcome), by mouth or by injection, is only used in hospital, after careful examination. Morphine may cause both colic and nausea.

Diarrhoea

Attention to dietary details improves this symptom. Codeine phosphate is also effective, but the most widely used antidiarrhoeal agent is diphenoxylate ("Lomotil," Searle). The small white tablets contain 2·5 mg diphenoxylate along with 0·025 mg atropine sulphate. Two tablets are taken 2 or 3 times per day, or as required. The drug decreases intestinal motility within 20 mins., and it does not give rise to the troublesome side-effects on vision and micturition that are associated with propantheline. There may be some dryness of the mouth.

Following resection of small intestine, irritation to the mucosa may result from the accumulation of fatty and other acids in the lumen. Calcium carbonate, in a daily dose of 15–30 gm, is said to be good in preventing diarrhoea from this cause (Le Veen *et al.*, 1967). A more popular explanation of diarrhoea after ileal resection is the presence of bile salts in the colon where they interfere with the normal reabsorption of water. Two bile salt binding agents, cholestyramine and lignin, have been tried in an attempt to reduce the quantity of unbound bile salts reaching the colon. Up to 16 gm of cholestyramine ("Questran," Bristol Myer) are required each day, given orally in divided doses. This anionic exchange resin certainly reduces the frequency of bowel action. The dose is large. Furthermore, cholestyramine may cause abdominal pain and it can precipitate acute obstruction when the lumen is already narrowed. It may interfere with vitamin D absorption (Thompson and Thompson, 1969). Cholestyramine treatment increases faecal fat excretion. Shuster *et al.* (1970) have successfully added the emulsifier polysorbate-80 ("Tween 80," Atlas Chemicals) to counteract the inefficient formation of micelles in the upper small intestine. If more than 100 cm of ileum have been removed, cholestyramine has less influence on bowel frequency (Hofmann and Poley, 1969). The author now restricts the use of cholestyramine to those patients whose diarrhoea fails to respond to other measures. Lignin (Therapharm, Ltd.), a hemi-cellulose prepared from wood, is more palatable than cholestyramine (Eastwood and Eriksson, 1970). However, it is less effective (Heaton *et al.*, 1971). The recommended dose varies between 6 gm and 10 gm per day. Faecal fat losses are not altered.

Kaolin preparations are sometimes used in Crohn's disease. By themselves they are unable to control severe diarrhoea, but like many of the agents listed, they are mostly used in conjunction with potent anti-inflammatory drugs.

Correction of Deficiencies

Fluid and Electrolytes
Severe dehydration and electrolyte depletion is seldom encountered in the early stages of Crohn's disease. They can appear during chronic illness, with profuse diarrhoea, sepsis and fistulae. In these ill patients intravenous therapy is necessary.

Sodium
Supplementary sodium may be given orally to patients with ulcerative colitis, but this is not necessary in Crohn's disease. If large losses have been sustained they are made good by the intravenous infusion of 0·9 per cent sodium chloride solution.

Potassium

Both Crohn's disease and its treatment with corticosteroids increase the loss of potassium. Such patients may need supplementary potassium, usually administered as either slow release tablets (8 m.Eq of K per tablet) or as effervescent tablets (12 mEq of K). From 2 to 6 tablets are taken daily for a short time. If the loss continues, preventative measures must be taken. These may include operation, in the preparation for which intravenous KCl, 1 gm per 500 ml of 5 per cent dextrose, is given. A depleted patient may be given up to 6 gm KCl in 24 hr, monitoring the ECG and serum concentration daily.

Calcium and Magnesium

Patients with steatorrhoea may benefit from additional calcium. The daily dose of calcium gluconate or lactate tablets is from 1–4 gm, either alone or combined with vitamin D. The serum calcium level must be checked at intervals. If there is evidence of hypomagnesaemia (p. 109), 4 ml of 50 per cent magnesium sulphate is taken orally. The intramuscular route can also be used but is painful.

Blood Formation

Hypochromic anaemia is common and responds to oral iron, e.g. ferrous sulphate, 200 mg tablet twice daily for 3 weeks or until the patient's haemoglobin is restored to an acceptable level. If one form of oral iron causes gastrointestinal irritation, another form such as ferrous fumarate or gluconate may be tried. It is not often necessary to resort to intramuscular iron ("Jectofer," Astra). With gross degrees of anaemia it is better to give a slow transfusion of packed red cells.

Many untreated patients with Crohn's disease do have a low serum folate level. During antibiotic treatment the level may be subnormal. However, it is by no means certain that they all need folic acid tablets (therapeutic dose 5 mg t.d.s.; for maintenance 0·3 mg per day). Should the low level persist in spite of the exhibition of anti-inflammatory drugs, the folic acid might reasonably be added. If the MCV or MCHC (p. 124) of the blood of any patient deviates from the normal range, the advice of a haematologist is obtained. Only a few patients who have widespread small intestinal disease or have had most of their ileum excised show vitamin B_{12} malabsorption. To replenish their body stores such patients are given 1,000 μg of hydroxocobalamin intramuscularly on alternate days over a 10 to 12 day period. Thereafter the same dose is injected once every 2 months.

Vitamins

The fat-soluble vitamins A, D and K may be deficient in patients with steatorrhoea. Strong calciferol tablets containing 50,000 units of vitamin D are available. It is more usual to give compound vitamin capsules, e.g. vitamin A 4,500 units plus vitamin D 450 units. When fruit and fresh vegetables are not being eaten, it is advisable for the patient to take ascorbic acid tablets, 250–500 mg per day.

Food Supplements

Patients who are unable or afraid to eat large solid meals can be helped by giving them concentrated food preparations. In 100 gm of Complan (Glaxo) there are 31 gm protein, 16 gm fat, 44 gm carbohydrate, plus electrolytes and vitamins. The powder can be added to ordinary dishes, made up as cup feeds or used in 20 per cent dilution for intragastric tube feeds. Casilan (Glaxo) is a whole protein powder, containing all the essential amino-acids; it may be incorporated in any dish made with milk or water, or may be sprinkled dry onto cold food.

Many Crohn's patients have or are on the borderline of getting steatorrhoea. It is inadvisable to give them extra fat. Their bile salt pool may be depleted and it is better for them to take whatever fat they can digest in the morning when there are more bile salts available than later on in the day. Medium chain triglycerides (MCT) are more easily digested and absorbed than conventional fat. They are less dependent on bile salts for emulsification, are more soluble and more rapidly hydrolysed than their long-chain counterparts. MCT oil (Mead Johnston) may be added to meat, salads or used in baking; the recommended intake is 15 ml thrice daily. Portagen powder (Mead Johnston) is composed of protein, carbohydrates, MCT and vitamins; one measuring cup (138 gm) supplies 640 calories. Any patient who needs these nutritional supplements should be seen by the dietitian. *Intragastric and Jejunostomy Tube Feeding:* These techniques of alimentation are rarely indicated in Crohn's disease. There is little point in pouring nutrients into the small intestine when it is known that there is diseased mucosa or a fistula a short distance downstream. It is very difficult to make up a feed which will not exacerbate the patient's bowel symptoms. Fat emulsions, e.g. Prosparol (B.D.H.), increase steatorrhoea, while concentrated carbohydrate or protein preparations are likely to make diarrhoea worse. If the correct composition can be found, tube feeds may be used to supplement whatever food an under-nourished patient is able to eat. Today when a patient with Crohn's disease is unable to take sufficient calories by mouth, it is more common to rely on intravenous feeding, either total or supplementary.

Intravenous Alimentation

Only a few patients with Crohn's disease require intravenous feeding. The concept of using total parenteral alimentation to provide complete rest for small intestine that is the site of very active inflammation is gaining ground. Very occasionally a patient first attends hospital having lost a great deal of weight and being unwilling to ingest an adequate diet—anorexia nervosa may be simulated. Such a patient will probably not tolerate a naso-gastric tube for intra-gastric feeding for any length of time. Consequently intravenous alimentation has to be resorted to, so that elective surgery can be performed on a better nourished patient. A more common indication for giving parenteral nutrients is when sepsis, fistula formation or breakdown of anastomoses follows operations for or recurrence of Crohn's disease. The nutritional status of some of these latter patients is grave. Furthermore, sepsis poses an ever-present danger of bacteraemia, and by increasing catabolism makes it very difficult for the patient to revert to a positive nitrogen balance and start to gain weight. In any programme of intravenous feeding, infection needs to be combated and abscesses drained as soon as possible if the maximum benefit is to be obtained.

Close supervision of intravenous alimentation is required and must be maintained for weeks on end. It is advisable to designate one member of the medical team who will be responsible throughout, not only for calculating the calorie intake and ensuring that it is given in the correct form, but also for assessing ordinary fluid and electrolyte requirements. The unfortunate patient is much more likely to be a 40–50 kg female rather than the traditional 70 kg male. However, because of the large deficits that have been incurred and the increased catabolism, a daily calorie intake of 2,500–3,000 calories is desirable.

Intravenous fat preparations and amino-acids interfere with the analyses in certain liver function tests and in haematological tests. Any anaemia should be corrected by transfusion before the intravenous alimentation regime is started. For daily electrolyte determinations, the intravenous drip should have been running on 5 per cent dextrose alone for 4 hours before a blood sample is drawn.

A large intravenous catheter is used, e.g. Intracath (Bardic); its tip should be in a major vein such as the superior vena cava. Strict aseptic precautions must be observed when inserting it and when changing infusion sets. Normally two sets are used in parallel, being joined together by a Y piece close to the catheter. If pyrexia develops, a blood culture is taken, the infusion is discontinued and the tip of the catheter is sent for bacteriological examination.

Fat is the richest source of calories, providing over 9 calories per gm. One litre of 20 per cent Intralipid (Vitrum*) should yield 2,000 calories. In practice 500 ml bottles are easier to handle. Modern fat emulsions are not irritant to the vein, but no pharmaceutical preparations can be added to them. Side-effects are rare, consisting of headache, backache, rigors and perhaps anaemia and coagulation defects (Walker and Johnston, 1971).

---

* Distributed by Paines and Byrne, Ltd., Greenford, Middlesex.

Amino-acids are more important for building body protein than for releasing calories. They are most useful when administered in the laevo-rotatory form and along with carbohydrate. One litre of 10 per cent Aminosol (Vitrum) yields 320 calories, while the same volume of synthetic amino-acids contained in 7 per cent Vamin (Vitrum) provide twice that number of calories. Magnesium is needed for protein synthesis.

A concentration of dextrose greater than 5 per cent is irritant to the veins, but the calorie content of the commonly used 5 per cent solution is low. Fructose is an alternative source of carbohydrate, rapidly metabolized in the liver. It has a tendency to increase urinary sodium and potassium losses, which must be watched. Fructose is often given in a 3·3 per cent Aminosol solution, along with a small quantity of ethyl alcohol, the mixture providing 875 calories per litre. Sorbitol, (Selpharm) a sugar alcohol, can be given in 30 per cent or 20 per cent solutions; weight for weight it has a slightly higher calorific value than dextrose or fructose.

Table I

Daily intravenous feeding for a 50 kg female with external fistulae

		Volume	Calories
I	Intralipid 20%	500 ml	1,000
	*Dextrose 5%	500 ml	100
II	Aminosol/Fructose/Ethanol	500 ml⎫	875
	Aminosol/Fructose/Ethanol	500 ml⎭	
III	Sorbitol 30%	500 ml	600
	*Dextrose 5%	500 ml	100
		3,000 ml	2,675

* Antibiotics, vitamins and KCl can be added to the dextrose solution. If they are not required, one 500 ml bottle of 10 per cent Intralipid may be substituted and provides 500 calories.

Most of these intravenous preparations are administered at the rate of 30 to 60 drops per minute. The composition of a typical intra-venous feeding programme is shown in Table I. Regular weighing of the patient provides a useful check on whether or not the intake is adequate.

Anti-inflammatory Agents

Drugs to kill or to arrest the proliferation of bacteria, to modify the inflammatory response to injury and to suppress immunopatho-logical reactions may be used alone or in combination. Crohn's disease patients who are in remission are given relatively small maintenance doses. During a relapse the dosage is increased and is kept at the higher level until the symptoms are brought under control once again. The ill-effects produced by the long-term administration of some of these drugs are considered in the final chapter of this book.

1. Antibiotics and Sulphonamide Compounds

These anti-bacterial substances do help to improve the symptoms in Crohn's disease. Pain, diarrhoea and general toxicity are all diminished. It is most improbable that any primary aetiological agent is being destroyed. A more likely explanation is that these drugs reduce the load of super-added infection that the damaged intestine has to contend with.

Ampicillin—This antibiotic is given in a dosage of 250 mg every 6 hours. The normal rule that a bacterial sensitivity test should be performed before starting treatment is not observed. After 3 to 5 days of ampicillin therapy some improvement often is apparent. The antibiotic may reasonably be given for a further week, but at the end of this time it must be reckoned to have achieved its greatest immediate effect on the flora of the small intestine. Continuance beyond this time is really suppression therapy—and it is not quite certain what is being suppressed. Bacteria may be rendered resistant to a valuable antibiotic, which then cannot be used should an emergency arise. In spite of these theoretical objections, ampicillin treatment has been maintained for 3 months and longer. The results of prolonged treatment are not known, and no double-blind trial has been carried out. Ampicillin frequently produces skin rashes.

Phthalylsulphathiazole and Sulphaguanide—These compounds are available in 500 mg tablets, the total daily dose being up to 8 gm. Patients may be willing to swallow the large number of tablets involved for a short time but are unlikely to do so for weeks on end. The tablets are relatively safe and can be taken with them by patients who are going on holidays abroad.

Sulphasalazine—Marketed as Salazopyrin* (Pharmacia), this azo compound of sulphapyridine and salicylic acid is the drug that has been most widely used in Crohn's disease. There is no agreement about its mode of action or effectiveness. A controlled clinical trial is in progress in Britain. It is doubtful if the effect of sulphasalazine is due to any antibacterial action (Cooke, 1969). During the last 10 years the majority of patients with Crohn's disease in Aberdeen have been given sulphasalazine at one time or another. It is the distinct clinical impression that the drug is beneficial in the more florid stages of the disease and safe for long-term treatment (Kyle, 1971).

Sulphasalazine is available in two forms—(i) plain large 0·5 gm tablets, and (ii) coated, ovoid En-tabs. The En-tabs are easier to

---

* Azulfidine in the United States of America.

swallow, and less likely to cause the nausea that a small proportion of patients complain of. During remissions two tablets are taken 2 or 3 times per day, and the treatment may continue for years; in an exacerbation 6–8 gm may be administered every 24 hours.

Apart from nausea, the other side-effects that are rarely seen include skin rashes and haemolytic anaemia. The latter condition could lead to excessive utilization of folate. However, the serum folate level may appear falsely low because sulphasalazine inhibits the growth of the test organism, *Lactobacillus casei*, that is used in the assay. Patients taking sulphasalazine should have their blood picture checked weekly for the first month. A urinary output of over 1,000 ml per 24 hours is advised.

2. Corticosteroids and Corticotrophin

The pharmacological action of corticosteroids in suppressing inflammatory reactions is useful in Crohn's disease. Hydrocortisone can be given systemically when the patient is unable to take anything by mouth. However, for most patients the steroid is given in tablet form, usually along with an antibiotic or sulphasalazine. Prednisone and prednisolone are the preparations in common use. The more powerful betamethasone has also been tried (Gill *et al.*, 1965) but it has not become popular. During severe attacks and in relapses 30–50 mg of prednisone are given each day for 2 weeks; thereafter the dose is gradually reduced to 5 or 10 mg per day. Dosage has to be varied according to the patient's weight and the clinical response. Clearly if 50 mg prednisone are given to a 50 kg female for several weeks serious side-effects will appear. On the other hand there is some doubt if 5 mg prednisone per day as maintenance therapy has any significant effect. Sparberg and Kirsner (1966) considered that 15 mg was the smallest dose that had any influence on the disease. The response to corticosteroids tends to be variable and unpredictable. Young patients with short histories do somewhat better than older patients. However, neither the mode of presentation nor the dosage of prednisone seems to influence the behaviour of Crohn's disease during the ensuing years. Some patients do not respond even to high doses of prednisone; after 2 weeks it is worth changing the treatment and trying corticotrophin instead.

When administered in high dosage, corticosteroids will diminish diarrhoea, reduce pain and lower the ESR. Watch must be kept for evidence of fluid retention, electrolyte disturbances and hypertension. Patients may develop psychotic problems, become osteoporotic, and have hyperglycaemia with glycosuria (Goldstein *et al.*, 1967). Potassium losses in the urine increase during cortisone therapy and there may be interference with calcium-vitamin D transport mechanisms in the small intestine. At St Mark's Hospital, steroids brought about considerable immediate improvement in approximately two-thirds of patients treated (Jones and Lennard-Jones, 1966). Unfortunately patients tended to relapse if the corticosteroids were discontinued. Three-quarters of the Birmingham patients treated with corticosteroids derived some short-term benefit (Cooke and Fielding, 1970). However, the steroid-treated group were twice as likely to come to surgery and had a mortality 4 times that of patients not given steroids. In Aberdeen, corticosteroids are used to help control initial attacks of Crohn's disease, or to reduce the activity of a severe relapse so that the patient may be prepared for definitive surgery. Small doses of prednisone are given, along with sulphasalazine, to patients who it is hoped can be kept symptom-free for a long time on medical treatment. Such patients should be issued with a card stating the type and dosage of the cortico-steroid they are receiving.

Children with Crohn's disease are liable to suffer from growth retardation, and the exhibition of corticosteroids may increase this tendency. Consequently it is better to treat children with corticotrophin, rather than give them prednisone. Corticotrophin gel is injected intra-muscularly, 40 or 80 units daily at the start, with up to 120 units for adults. Later the frequency of injections is reduced. Synacthen (Ciba) is an alternative preparation, 1 mg being injected twice weekly. Assays of pituitary gonadotrophin in the urine are of no value in determining the response to corticosteroid or corticotrophin therapy (Crean, 1967).

Corticosteroids are also used locally, as suppositories or retention enemata. It is doubtful if suppositories containing prednisone can affect more than the distal third of the rectum. Predsol retention enemata (Glaxo), self-administered each evening for a week, do seem to bring about some improvement in Crohn's disease of the colon. The course may have to be repeated. Local applications of corticosteroid preparations to aphthous ulcers in the mouth have not been successful, there being no significant difference in the incidence or duration of ulceration (MacPhee *et al.*, 1968). Appreciable amounts of steroids can be absorbed into the systemic circulation during topical therapy.

Immunosuppression

Radiotherapy
At the time when it was first used in Crohn's disease (van Patter *et al.*, 1954) it was probably not appreciated that local radiotherapy could suppress an immune reaction. The results were variable and the dis-advantages not inconsiderable. Bargen (1957) believed that it helped a few advanced cases, but no proper trial has been conducted. Fruin *et al.* (1967) were very doubtful about the advisability of using radio-therapy. No patient in north-east Scotland has been treated by this method. Local irradiation has been of value in transplantation. If an

immunopathological aetiology for Crohn's disease is definitely established, there may be a case for re-considering the use of modern radiotherapy techniques as an adjunct to other forms of treatment, for
example on a localized recurrence in a patient who already has had
numerous operations.

Nitrogen Mustard

Winkelman and Brown (1965) reported on the treatment of 13 patients
with Crohn's disease who were given a total dose of up to 20 mg of
nitrogen mustard intravenously over 6 days, along with corticotrophin.
Nine patients responded satisfactorily, 6 of them having uncomplicated
disease. The treatment failed in 4 patients, 2 of whom developed
acute obstruction and 2 perforated. The late results in this small
series of patients are not known. The intravenous administration of
nitrogen mustard requires careful supervision, and with the introduction of azathioprine, which is taken by mouth, use of nitrogen mustard
has been abandoned.

Azathioprine

In 1972 the exact place of azathioprine (Imuran, Burroughs Wellcome)
in the treatment of Crohn's disease is not clear. The drug is most
commonly given as 100 mg (2 tablets) per day, or in a dose of 2 mg per
kg body weight. Up to 5 mg per kg have been used for short periods,
together with prednisolone, the dose being reduced after several weeks
to a maintenance level. An alternative schedule is to give the higher
dosage for 5 days, followed by corticosteroids for 2 days, and then
repeat the sequence. White cell counts must be carried out twice weekly
on starting azathioprine, and later the blood is checked every 2 weeks.

The first report from St George's Hospital, London (Brooke *et al.*,
1969) described 6 patients with advanced disease; 4 had troublesome
fistulae. All cases had proved refractory to other forms of medical
and surgical treatment. When given 4 mg azathioprine per kg body
weight for 10 days, and 2 mg per kg thereafter, all these ill patients
markedly improved. The fistulae all dried up and 5 out of the 6 patients
returned to work. A transient leucopenia was common and as the ESR
remained elevated, it appeared that the activity of the Crohn's disease
persisted in spite of the symptomatic improvement. The follow-up
period was very short.

A double-blind crossover trial on 14 patients was conducted by
Rhodes *et al.* (1970). According to the patient's estimate of the result
there was little to choose between the placebo and the azathioprine, and
the latter certainly caused leucopenia occasionally and arthralgia in
one case. A second report (Rhodes *et al.*, 1971) advised caution in the
use of azathioprine. Other workers (Jones *et al.*, 1969; Drucker and
Jeejeebhoy, 1970; Kasper *et al.*, 1970; Arden Jones, 1971) have reported

small numbers of patients treated with azathioprine. Between 40 per cent and 80 per cent of the patients improved; the 100 per cent success rate of the first study has never again been achieved. Brown and Achkar (1970) felt the best results were obtained when azathioprine was given together with sulphasalazine and corticosteroids; they did not advocate its use in acute attacks. In the 9 severe cases from Toronto (Drucker and Jeejeebhoy, 1970) it was 4 to 9 weeks before there was any evidence of improvement—less pain, reduction in diarrhoea and gain in weight. Benefit was maximal at 24 weeks.

Willoughby *et al.* (1971) have performed a controlled double-blind trial of azathioprine over a trial period, also of 24 weeks. Acutely ill patients receiving azathioprine went into remission much sooner than those getting the placebo. Ninety per cent of the former group remained in remission up to the end of the 24 weeks, whereas 72 per cent of the placebo group had to be withdrawn from the trial because they relapsed. Most of these patients did take prednisolone at some time. Furthermore, 24 weeks represents less than 1 per cent of the life expectancy of a young adult—one of the major unanswered problems at the present time is how long to continue with azathioprine treatment.

In a second report from St George's Hospital, Brooke *et al.* (1970) stated that 6 out of 24 patients had done badly or failed to respond. They concluded that azathioprine worked best in early colonic disease, with recurrent lesions and when there were fistulae. They did not find it helpful when there was ileitis plus a mass.

The Aberdeen experience has been similar to that of Papp *et al.* (1971), namely that approximately 50 per cent of patients are helped significantly by azathioprine treatment. During two years, 16 patients aged between 20 years and 77 years, were given courses of azathioprine, alone or with prednisone. The dose was 100 mg per day in most instances. One patient had to discontinue treatment because of a white cell count persistently below 3,000 per cu.mm, and it was doubtful if another elderly lady took her tablets regularly. Two patients complained of nausea. Twelve of the 14 patients who persisted with azathioprine for more than 4 weeks derived some benefit, particularly as regards their diarrhoea. Ten patients made modest gains in weight, although their serum proteins tended to fall, the decrease being in the globulin fraction (from mean of 3·9 mg to a mean of 3·1 mg per 100 ml). Comparable barium X-ray films before and after treatment were available in 4 patients; they showed no evidence of regression of the disease. The greatest disappointment was the failure of fistulae to heal. One external abdominal wall fistula closed for 3 weeks and then commenced to discharge again. Azathioprine had no effect on another external fistula. Only 1 out of 3 ano-rectal fistulae remained healed for more than 6 weeks.

One unresolved worry about the prolonged administration of

azathioprine is the possibility that sarcomas or other mesenchymal tumours may finally appear. Thirty-seven transplant patients given immunosuppressive drugs have developed such neoplasms (Starzl *et al.*, 1970). Admittedly the antigenic challenge of a transplanted organ could be responsible, and may be very intense (the 7 metres of small intestine could constitute a sizeable challenge). Neoplasms can also arise in patients receiving azathioprine for diseases with an immuno-pathological basis (Sharpstone *et al.*, 1969). So far no report of a drug-induced neoplasm in Crohn's disease has appeared.

There is a slight danger that a child may be born with congenital defects if the father was taking azathioprine at the time of fertilization, or the mother was taking it during the early stages of pregnancy.

It is interesting to note that among their transplant patients the Denver workers (Penn *et al.*, 1970) had 11 cases of severe inflammation of the colon. Whether the inflammation was caused by the original disease, the transplant or the immunosuppressive drugs is not known.

Antilymphocytic Serum

At the present time the antilymphocytic serum (ALS) available consists of a complex mixture of antibodies and non-specific proteins. Nearly all the antilymphocytic antibodies are in the IgG fraction. They are potent and highly specific immunosuppressants. With further refinements in their preparation and separation it may be possible to use them in the treatment of Crohn's disease. There is less likelihood of secondary infection than with immunosuppressive drugs (James, 1970), but the risk of late tumour formation is not eliminated (Zipp and Kountz, 1971).

By one or more of the lines of medical treatment outlined above and with constant attention to nutrition, it is possible to keep many patients with Crohn's disease in tolerable health for long periods of time. When most of the intestine is diseased and when recurrence takes place after radical resection, medical measures are the only form of treatment possible. However, in young patients with localized lesions the decision about treatment is less easy to make. In the absence of mechanical complications such patients can be kept comfortable on a medical regime. Nevertheless there are certain drawbacks. As well as the serious side-effects of some drugs, obstruction and perforation remain ever-present hazards. At the start of medical treatment the doctor knows the very large number of drugs that will have to be taken, and that probably the patient will have to remain under surveillance for the remainder of his or her life. If they were in possession of this knowledge, many patients would opt for the alternative to this type of medicated survival, namely surgical treatment.

References

Arden Jones, R. (1971), *Proc. r. Soc. Med.*, **64**, 171.

Bargen, J. A. (1957), *Ann. intern. Med.*, **47**, 875.

Brooke, B. N., Hoffmann, D. C. and Swarbrick, E. T. (1969), *Lancet*, **2**, 612.

Brooke, B. N., Javett, S. L. and Davison, O. W. (1970), *Lancet*, **2**, 1050.

Brown, C. H. and Achkar, E. (1970), *Am. J. Gastroent.*, **54**, 363.

Cooke, W. T. and Fielding, J. F. (1970), *Gut*, **11**, 921.

Cooke, E. M. (1969), *Gut*, **10**, 565.

Crean, G. P. (1967), *Gut*, **7**, 597.

Drucker, W. R. and Jeejeebhoy, K. N. (1970), *Ann. Surg.*, **172**, 618.

Eastwood, M. A. and Eriksson, S. (1970), *Gut*, **11**, 370.

Fielding, J. F. and Cooke, W. T. (1969), *Gut*, **10**, 1054.

Fruin, R. C., Miree, J. and Littman, A. (1967), *Gastroenterology*, **52**, 134.

Gill, A. M., Otaki, A. T., Daly, J. R. and Spencer-Peet, J. R. (1965), *Brit. med. J.*, **2**, 29.

Goldstein, M. J., Gelzayd, E. A. and Kirsner, J. B. (1967), *Trans. Amer. Acad. Ophth. Otol.*, **82**, 254.

Heaton, K. W., Heaton, S. T. and Barry, R. E. (1971), *Scand. J. Gastroent.*, **6**, 281.

Hofmann, A. F. and Poley, J. R. (1969), *Gastroenterology*, **56**, 1168.

James, K. (1970), *Proc. r. Soc. Med.*, **63**, 951.

Jones, F. A., Brown, P., Lennard-Jones, J. E., Jones, J. H. and Milton-Thompson, G. J. (1969), *Lancet*, **2**, 795.

Jones, J. H. and Lennard-Jones, J. E. (1966), *Gut*, **7**, 181.

Kasper, H., Zimmerman, H. D. and Nagels, D. (1970), *Deutsch. med. Wschr.*, **95**, 1261.

Kyle, J. (1971), *Ulster med. J.*, **40**, 59.

Le Veen, H. H., Borek, B., Axelrod, R. D. and Johnson, A. (1967), *Surg. Gynec. Obstet.*, **124**, 766.

MacPhee, I. T., Sircus, W., Farmer, E. D., Harkness, R. A. and Cowley, G. C. (1968), *Brit. med. J.*, **2**, 147.

Papp, J. P., Bull, F. E. and Watson, D. W. (1971), *Gastroenterology*, **60**, 705.

Penn, I., Brettschneider, L., Simpson, K., Martin, A. and Stazl, T. E. (1970), *Arch. Surg.* (*Chicago*), **100**, 61.

Rhodes, J., Bainton, D., and Beck, P. (1970), *Lancet*, **2**, 1142.

Rhodes, J., Bainton, D., Beck, P. and Campbell, H. (1971), *Lancet*, **2**, 1273.

Sharpstone, P., Ogg, C. S. and Cameron, S. J. (1969), *Brit. med. J.*, **2**, 535.

Shuster, F., Spot, R. C. and Jacobs, M. N. (1970), *Amer. J. Digest. Dis.*, **15**, 353.

Sparberg, M. and Kirsner, J. B. (1966), *Amer. J. Digest. Dis.*, **11**, 865.

Starzl, T. E., Porter, K. A., Andrew, G., Halgrimson, G., Hurwitz, R., Giles, G., Terasaki, P. I., Lilly, J. and Putnam, C. W. (1970), *Ann. Surg.*, **172**, 437.

Thompson, W. G. and Thompson, G. R. (1969), *Gut*, **10**, 717.

Van Patter, W. N., Bargen, J. A., Dockerty, M. B., Feldman, W. H., Mayo, C. W. and Waugh, J. M. (1954), *Gastroenterology*, **26**, 347.

Walker, W. F. and Johnston, I. D. A. (1971). *The Metabolic Basis of Surgical Care.* London: Heinemann Medical Books.

Willoughby, J. M. T., Kumar, P. F., Beckett, J. and Dawson, A. M. (1971), *Lancet*, **2**, 944.

Winkelman, E. I. and Brown, C. H. (1965), *Cleveland Clinic Quart.*, **32**, 165.

Zipp, P. and Kountz, S. L. (1971), *Amer. J. Surg.*, **122**, 204.

Chapter IX
Surgical Treatment

The type of operation recommended for the common form of Crohn's disease in the terminal ileum has changed several times during the 40 years since the disease was first described. To begin with radical resection was practised but in 1932 the mortality was unacceptably high. Simple short-circuiting procedures were rapidly followed by relapse or recurrence of the disease and so were abandoned. The staff of the Mount Sinai Hospital, New York, then developed the operation of short-circuit with exclusion to completely divert the faecal stream away from the damaged lower ileum. This operation had a low mortality and many external fistulae dried up, but it was never fully accepted by the protagonists of resection. With the introduction of the sulphonamides and antibiotics, intestinal surgery became progressively safer, and the pendulum of surgical opinion swung back in favour of resection, when feasible, as being the treatment of choice in chronic Crohn's disease. By the time that Crohn's disease of the colon was recognized, surgical techniques for dealing with ulcerative colitis had been perfected and were immediately applicable to the transmural type of colonic inflammation.

Indications for Operation

The presence of a major complication constitutes the clearest indication for surgical intervention in several gastrointestinal diseases, for example duodenal ulceration and diverticulitis. Acute complications of Crohn's disease, such as perforation and complete obstruction, likewise require surgical treatment. In about 5 per cent of cases it is clinically impossible to differentiate between acute suppurative appendicitis and an acute presentation of Crohn's disease, so that laparotomy is essential.

However in the majority of patients the first operation for Crohn's disease is an elective one. There is time to consider and weigh up a number of factors, not the least of which is the nuisance and long-term hazards to the patient of prolonged medical treatment. The hopes and fears of the patient must be given proper consideration (Kyle, 1964). The main indications for elective surgery in chronic Crohn's disease are set out in Table 1.

It is never easy to define "failure of medical therapy". In the first place the physician and surgeon together must be satisfied that the regime prescribed was both adequate and was adhered to by the patient. The various possible combinations of drugs given in Chapter VIII should

Table 1
Indications for elective operation
1. Failure of adequate medical therapy.
2. Inability to enjoy life, stunting of growth.
3. Localized quiescent disease.
4. Subacute intestinal obstruction.
5. External fistulae.
6. Abdominal mass.
7. Persistent anaemia, hypoproteinaemia.
8. Chronic systemic complications.

have been tried and full nutritional support provided. The symptoms of a few patients may continue to get worse even when they are on high dosage drug therapy and it may be felt that surgery offers the only hope of halting the progress of the disease; the prognosis is not good. Luckily this sequence of events is unusual. More often medical treatment results in considerable improvement, but one or two symptoms persist to an extent that cannot be ignored. There may be diarrhoea 3 or 4 times per day, or the patient remains underweight although taking supplements and eating as much as she can. After 3–6 months all concerned gradually realize the medical therapy has not produced the full remission that had been hoped for.

Particularly in young patients, inability to actually enjoy life and to develop normally constitute a valid indication for surgery, although it is an indication that may be difficult to appreciate at the time. These patients, often young girls, are small, pale, poorly developed and over-protected by anxious relatives, who for years have fed them pills to keep them free from distressing symptoms. These patients may be regarded as therapeutic successes, but they are being denied the happy, exciting life of a normal teenager. Surgery may offer them this latter prospect.

In many patients there is more than one indication for operation present. This is true of quiescent disease and stenoses giving rise to subacute obstruction. The surgeons at Mount Sinai Hospital used to like to wait if possible until the disease was "burnt out" before undertaking an elective operation (Garlock, 1967). It is the author's belief that patients who go into remission spontaneously or as a result of medical therapy and who remain well for a period of months do better following surgery than those operated on in an active and uncontrolled phase of their disease. With attempted repair and fibrosis, the lumen may become uncomfortably small. It is better to perform an elective resection in a fit patient rather than to wait until obstruction forces surgical intervention in a patient who is then ill.

Even when one or two episodes of subacute obstruction settle with non-operative treatment, it is clear for mechanical reasons that they will recur until the surgeon fashions an adequate passage for the intestinal contents. Less than 10 per cent of all chronic cases of Crohn's

disease have their first operation because of obstruction (de Dombal
et al., 1971). However, it is a much more common indication for second
and subsequent interventions.

Personal and economic considerations rather than strictly surgical
indications for resection may exist in patients with inactive disease
confined to a short length of the bowel. A man, otherwise well, who
has a palpable lump in his lower abdomen may wish to be rid of the
abnormality. Seamen, patients working overseas or in the Armed
Forces in general are better treated surgically rather than medically.

External fistulae frequently follow incision of a lower abdominal
mass thought to be an appendix abscess. Such fistulae are a considerable
nuisance, although not disabling. They show little tendency to heal up
on their own. An abdominal mass associated with obstructive signs in
an older patient may well be diagnosed as a colonic neoplasm if time
does not permit barium studies to be performed. An exploratory
laparotomy could justifiably be carried out.

Occasionally a patient is encountered in whom there is considerable
difficulty in keeping the blood picture normal although other symptoms
and signs of Crohn's disease respond readily to medical treatment.
Oedema due to hypoproteinaemia is another manifestation which in
a few Aberdeen patients has not subsided as expected. Excision of the
ulcerated intestine produces a speedy recovery.

Skin, eye and joint complications by no means always vanish when
abdominal symptoms subside in response to the physician's efforts.
Admittedly attacks of inflammation in these other structures become
less frequent and less severe, but they may not disappear completely
until all diseased intestine has been removed.

Timing of Operation

The timing of elective surgery is of some importance. Ideally the
patient's disease should be in remission, all gross deficiencies should
have been corrected and he should be starting to gain weight. With
intensive drug therapy, the ESR often falls to less than half the reading
recorded in an acute attack. When this favourable state is reached and
before obstructive signs develop, the operation is performed. There is
nothing to be gained by further delay once conservative therapy has
shown its full effect and is unable to produce further improvement. As
Crohn (1957) has said: ". . . irresolute marking time merely prolongs
the painful and debilitating aspects of the disease; it creates often an
unhappy state of mind in the patient who lives suspended in doubt
having been told that operation is nevertheless the eventual solution of
his illness".

Krause (1971) has suggested that a trial should be conducted,
operating on cases alternately early and late in the course of their
disease. However, the best time to operate cannot be determined by the

calendar and the author would not support adherence to any rigid rule. Each patient has to be considered individually. When possible surgery is performed when the disease is quiescent and the patient is fit. The gloomy prospect of life-long steroid therapy in young patients may prompt rather earlier intervention, while middle-aged patients may be more willing to tolerate continuance with and changes in medical treatment.

Pre-Operative Preparation

The immediate pre-operative preparations advocated in Aberdeen are relatively simple. Neomycin, 1 gm twice or three times daily, is given for 2 days. A simple enema is administered the day before operation to clear the colon of any faecal masses and more especially of any residual barium; the enema may have to be repeated. A loaded colon at operation increases the risk of ileus and wound sepsis afterwards (Barker *et al.*, 1971). A blood sample is sent for cross-matching, and the transfusion service is requested to have 2 units of blood (1,000 ml) ready should need arise. In practice blood loss during operation is mostly small. On the morning of operation a naso-gastric tube is passed in order to keep the stomach empty. The anaesthetist must be warned if the patient has taken corticosteroids during the preceding 6 months. When a dissection within the pelvis is anticipated, a small Foley catheter is inserted into the bladder in the theatre before the operation commences.

Resection of Ileum

The operation described in this section is applicable to 60 per cent of cases with disease localized to the terminal ileum. The mucosa of the right colon is an important site of water absorption and as much of it as possible should be conserved to diminish the risk of diarrhoea after operation. When caecum and colon are healthy, the bowel is transected a short distance beyond the ileo-caecal valve, but on the ileal side it is divided well above the main mass. The operation is completed by an end-to-end anastomosis, giving a virtually normal anatomical configuration and a good physiological result. When Crohn's disease also involves the contiguous parts of caecum and ascending colon, the latter is divided at a more distal level. If the entire ascending colon is diseased, the operation can be extended to include all the large bowel that is removed in a classical right hemicolectomy.

The abdomen is opened through a lower right paramedian incision. In a thin female with a mobile mass the incision does not usually need to be more than 10 cm long, but there should be no hesitation in extending it so as to gain unimpeded access to the abdominal contents. A little free peritoneal fluid is often noticed in acute or complicated cases. The thickened ileum is seen at once in many patients; in others it has to be drawn up out of the pelvis. In a small number of patients the mass is adherent to some deep and fixed structure, and can only be displayed by packing other coils of intestine over to the left side or into the upper part of the peritoneal cavity.

The diseased ileum is swollen and its serosa is injected and has lost its normal sheen. Some parts look whitish and rough, especially in long-standing lesions. Not uncommonly the fat of the mesentery attempts to encircle the circumference so that only the anti-mesenteric border is clearly seen. The lesion usually extends proximally from the ileo-caecal valve for 15–30 cms and there may be evidence of subacute obstruction in the middle portion of the ileum. Classically the mesentery is grossly thickened (up to 3 cm) and oedematous, but this is by no means always the case. The mesentery may be thin and readily transilluminable. Some degree of lymph node enlargement is present in the majority of patients. The mesenteric nodes can be as large as a walnut. It is necessary to take a careful look at their arrangement and distribution in order to decide the correct line along which to divide the mesentery.

Having determined the state of affairs in the right, lower abdomen the remainder of the gastrointestinal tract must be inspected and palpated from end to end, looking for a skip lesion. Widespread in-volvement of most of the intestine is, of course, immediately apparent. It is not unusual to find one or two skip lesions within a few centimetres of the main mass and they can be removed in continuity with it. A skip lesion is often short, 3–5 cm in length, and may have a rather smaller diameter than the adjacent, presumably normal, although possibly dilated bowel.

The colour of skip lesions is either purple or blanched and on pal-pation they have a cartilaginous consistency. It is sometimes easier to feel than to see a skip lesion. Not all lesions are in the distal ileum; there may be an isolated one in mid-jejunum or near the splenic flexure of the colon. It is for this reason that the examination of the gastro-intestinal tract has to be carried out in such a thorough manner. At this stage the gall-bladder is examined to see if it contains gall-stones (page 134) and a biopsy may be taken from the liver edge (page 131).

Once the extent of the disease is known the decision must be taken whether or not to proceed with resection. When most of the ileum (or more than 50 per cent of the small intestine) is clearly involved, there must be grave doubts about the efficacy of a radical operation. Patients can survive on 50 cm of jejunum but they do not enjoy the experience. All the relevant facts in the patient's history have to be rapidly weighed in the balance—duration, types of drugs given, number of earlier operations and complications and the therapeutic options still open to the clinician. In general, massive resection of the greater part of the small intestine is not advised. Fortunately, in the majority of patients the disease is localized and there is no hesitation in proceeding to resection.

Wound towels are laid along the sides of the incision, the remainder of the intestine is packed off, away from the field of resection, and a self-retaining retractor is put in position and opened.

Technique of Resection

With Crohn's disease confined to the terminal ileum, the aim is to remove the main mass along with 15–20 cm of healthy intestine on the proximal side and the smallest possible length of ascending colon on the distal side. The amount of mesentery removed is immaterial, provided that the main superior mesenteric blood vessels remain intact.

Adequate mobilization is essential so that the resection can be performed outside the abdominal wall. The parietal peritoneum below and lateral to the caecum and the commencement of the ascending colon is incised. The terminal ileum and caecum are drawn forward as they are separated by blunt dissection from the structures lying behind. Care has to be taken not to start bleeding from ovarian (or spermatic) vessels when they are being swept clear of the main mass. The right ureter is identified; a warm moist pack is laid over it and the adjacent raw surface while the resection proceeds.

The inflamed ileum may be loosely adherent to a nearby loop of intestine, often the sigmoid colon, or to uterus and Fallopian tube. In such circumstances the ileal mass can be pinched off the other viscus, oozing from the surface of the latter soon stopping under a warm pack. When it is the adjacent loop of ileum that is adherent, it is wiser to include it in the resected specimen. With dense adhesions behind and below, sharp dissection is likely to be needed. It is at this point that accurate judgment is required. Is it wise to persist with a sharp and rather blind dissection which may damage ureter, iliac vessels and other vital structures? Would it not be safer to choose the less heroic operation of short-circuit with exclusion, even though the long-term results in some cases are less satisfactory than those of resection? The over-riding consideration must be to leave the patient no worse off after the operation than she was before it.

When the main mass, perhaps along with one or two adjacent skip lesions and an adherent loop of ileum has been mobilized, the point where the ileum will be divided is selected. It should be in healthy intestine, 15–20 cm proximal to the upper visible limit of disease. The point is marked with a small Babcock tissue forceps. The ascending colon will be transected immediately above the ileo-caecal valve (Fig. 1). The leaf of mesentery is now inspected to determine along what line it will be divided.

Division of the Mesentery

The correct line to follow is the safest line. The chief danger with a very thick mesentery is that an unseen artery slips backwards out of a ligature and gives rise to a large haematoma in the base of the mesentery, which may be very difficult to control. The importance of conserving the main trunk of the superior mesenteric artery has already been mentioned. Undoubtedly the shortest route is the line between the Babcock's forceps on the ileum and the beginning of the ascending colon, which cuts across the right, lower part of the mesentery. If this line crosses a

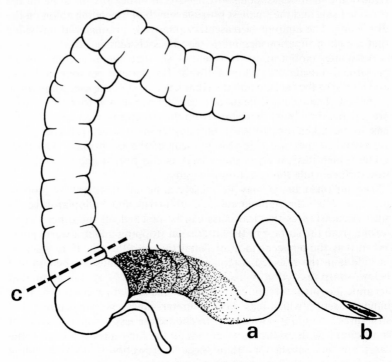

FIG. 1. Resection of terminal ileum for Crohn's disease. The length of normal ileum removed (*a* to *b*) with the specimen is 20 cm. The colon is transected along line *c*.

cluster of large juicy glands it is much safer to take the longer, more tedious route close to the intestinal wall rather than to attempt to include the nodes by following a more central course. It has been stated that radical extirpation of diseased bowel plus nodes produces better results than more limited resections (Wenckert *et al.*, 1970). Even if this is true, the improvement in the prognosis is probably accounted for by dividing the ileum at a higher level and not by removal of all big lymph nodes. Once nodes are macroscopically enlarged almost certainly there are microscopic changes much further afield. There seems little justification for expecting a cure to be achieved by the surgeon simply removing nodes that he sees are enlarged. Some patients have nodes close to the diseased ileum and another cluster situated basally; it is possible to pass safely between these two groups.

With a mesentery that is not unduly thick, the terminal ileo-colic part of the mesenteric artery can usually be seen in the ileo-caecal angle. When caecum and colon are healthy, swelling of the ileal mesentery may not extend into the angle. The blood vessels can be under-run with an aneurysm needle, ligated with silk or linen thread and divided. Other vessels supplying the affected zone can be seen on the front surface or by trans-illuminating the leaf of a thin mesentery, and they are secured individually.

When the mesentery is grossly thickened it is divided by a clamping and cutting technique, proceeding cautiously all the time. The author uses Mayo's haemostats (7 in; 17·5 cm long) in pairs, each bite of juicy tissue not being more than 1·5 cm. If there is any possibility of a ligature slipping, the tissue held in the more central haemostat is transfixed before being ligated with unabsorbable thread. As the wall of the intestine is approached, fine haemostats (Dunhills) are used to catch small pieces of fatty tissue or blood vessels. At least 1 cm of ileal and of colonic wall should be cleared of fat, appendices epiploicae, vessels and other impedimenta right round the entire circumference at the points where they are to be divided. For a good anastomosis it is vital that the surgeon can clearly see the muscle in the bowel wall that he knows will hold his stitches securely. A few extra minutes spent clearing the bowel ends may save the patient weeks or months spent in hospital afterwards because of a leaking anastomosis.

The Anastomosis
A "dirty" or "danger" towel is positioned around the abdominal incision. If the ileum is not dilated it must be cut obliquely at the expense of the anti-mesenteric border so that the long axis of the opening is approximately the same length as the diameter of the ascending colon above the caecum. Pairs of narrow-bladed Schoemaker crushing clamps are placed at the edge of the cleared band of intestinal wall that is nearer to the diseased ileum. The clamps are put on transversely across the start of the ascending colon, their points centrally; the clamps on the ileum are mostly at 45° across the long axis. The bowel is then divided at both places between the pairs of Schoemaker clamps, using either a scalpel or cutting diathermy point, and the specimen is removed. If oedema is obvious in the cut edge of the intestine, it suggests that it is unhealthy.

When the bowel has been properly mobilized the anastomosis can be performed outside the abdominal wall. The handles of the two remaining clamps are approximated, to appose the cut ends of ileum and colon. Care is taken that neither end has become twisted. Because of the bevel on the ileum, it may appear rather angulated. However, once the anastomosis is completed, with some compensatory flexion medially of the colon, the angulation largely disappears.

Outer stitches of black silk (Ethicon No. 333) through the sero-muscular layers are now inserted on the mesenteric and anti-mesenteric borders to draw the ends together. They are tied, and held in haemo-stats to act as stay stitches. With the blades of the clamps rolled slightly away from each other, one or two more posterior, interrupted stitches may be inserted to ensure that the length of the opening on the ileal side is the same as that in the colon. Soft occlusion clamps are now placed across both pieces of bowel about 3 cm clear of the crushing clamps, which are then removed.

The sides of the crushed fringe of tissue are teased apart. Any faecal material in the lumen is gently swabbed away, using pledgets soaked in a dilute antiseptic such as Savlon (ICI) or Dettol (Reckitt & Colman). It is important for the surgeon to get a clear view of the mucosa for a distance of about 2 cm into either end, particularly on the ileal side. He is looking for any signs of inflammation or ulceration, and especially for tiny punctate, "apthoid" ulcers (Morson, 1971). If any are located it means that resection has not been sufficiently radical, and a further 5 cm of ileum must be removed and the inspection then repeated.

Sections of ileal wall examined by the frozen section technique are frequently difficult to interpret, although when in doubt about the proximal ileal end, Wallensten (1971) has found this examination useful. Most British surgeons rely on inspection. It is difficult to decide just how far back further 5 cm resections should go. When necessary 2 or 3 segments can be removed but there comes a point when, with the proximal end still looking unhealthy, it may be more realistic to consider that the whole small intestine is pathological. In such circum-stances radical surgery is not the correct treatment. The surgeon then has to fashion an anastomosis, one side of which is unhealthy; the chance of a leak afterwards is considerable.

Starting on the anti-mesenteric border, the inner continuous stitch of 00 chromic catgut (Ethicon No. 441) is inserted, Fig. 2. A locking type of stitch is used along the back wall, changing to an inverting stitch for the inner corner and anterior layer. The exact type of stitch used is not very important. What is crucial is that the surgeon should see precisely where the needle goes every time. The atraumatic catgut needle goes through all coats, firmly uniting the serosal surfaces of the two ends. The stitches should be about 3 mm apart and, where they are seen on the back wall of the anastomosis, they should be 3 mm back from the free edge of the mucosa. It is highly dangerous to insert stitches blindly, hoping for the best and not knowing for certain that they have gone through the correct layers. Particular care must be

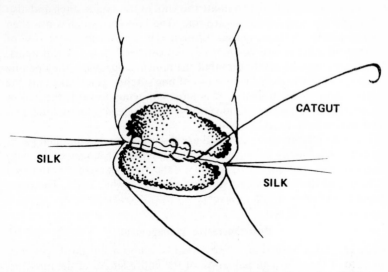

FIG. 2. Detail of anastomosis between ileum and ascending colon. While the line is steadied by traction on the outer, interrupted silk stitches, an inner continuous, locked catgut stitch is inserted.

taken to accurately infold the mesenteric end of the suture line; leaks are wont to occur at this point.

After completing the inner catgut layer, the surgeon puts in a series of interrupted silk stitches to turn in the anterior line of the anastomosis (Fig. 3). A small purse-string type stitch, with two sero-muscular bites on

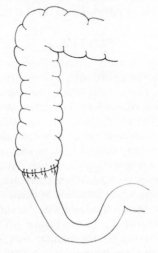

FIG. 3. The completed ileo-colic anastomosis.

each side, can be used to invaginate the knot of the catgut stitch and also the mesenteric end of the suture line. The two stay stitches are then used to rotate the anastomosis through 180° so that the back row of interrupted stitches can be inserted, the stitches being 3–4 mm apart. After checking with the fingers that the lumen is adequate, the opening in the mesentery is closed by a series of fine stitches which take only the anterior layer of peritoneum. It is most annoying, towards the end of the operation, to prick a blood vessel with a carelessly placed stitch and get a haematoma in the mesentery.

The dirty instruments and towel are discarded, and abdominal packs are removed. Finally haemostasis is checked and a Sterivac drain, with its inner end split for 6 cm, is laid in the right paracolic gutter and brought out through a small stab incision in the iliac fossa. The paramedian incision is closed in layers.

Post-Operative Management

Recovery after resection is remarkably smooth in most patients. Because of the thorough palpation of the entire length of the intestine, peristaltic activity may be slow to return. Fluid and electrolytes are continued intravenously. Once bowel sounds are heard on abdominal auscultation 15 ml of water are given hourly by mouth. The nasogastric tube is removed about this time if aspirates are low, and the intravenous infusion can be stopped the following day. Patients who had been on corticosteroids before operation must continue with them afterwards, the dose being tapered off over the next week or two. During the first 48 hours a little serous fluid or lymph may come from the drain, which is gradually shortened and removed. Most patients who had uncomplicated disease are able to return home on the 10th postoperative day.

Skip Lesions

One or two short skip lesions which are close to the inflamed terminal loop of ileum are removed along with it. When there is an isolated skip lesion in the jejunum, particularly if it is stenotic in character, it probably should be resected. About 6 cm of normal intestine on each side of it are also removed. The alternative is to short-circuit the obstructing lesion. However, when there is no evidence of obstruction, it is by no means certain that anything should be done. Several Aberdeen patients remain well although a jejunal skip lesion was left untouched at the time of ileal resection some years ago. When there are numerous skip areas it is logical to regard the whole intestine as diseased and not to attempt radical extirpation. In these circumstances the surgeon's main concern is to prevent acute obstruction in the future. One or two skip lesions may have to be by-passed. If the patient was suffering large faecal losses of blood and protein beforehand, it may still be justifiable to resect the terminal ileum. Once the possibility of mechanical complications has been circumvented, reliance is placed on immunosuppressants and antibiotics to keep the Crohn's disease in the upper small intestine under control.

Contact involvement of the sigmoid colon poses a different problem. The mucosal surface at the point of adherence can be seen and kept under observation with a colonoscope, or in a small patient, with a sigmoidoscope. In many patients in whom the adhesion can be broken down by pinching the ileal mass off it, nothing further need be done to the sigmoid colon, provided the wall feels supple. Regrettably, it is not unusual to find that the sigmoid wall is almost as thick and rigid as that of the ileum. It is involved by Crohn's disease. Sigmoid resection is desirable. This can be carried out by an open technique with immediate end-to-end anastomosis in a patient whose general condition is good. In a poor-risk patient a Paul-Mickulicz type of resection is performed. The colostomy is closed a few weeks later, and the result is satisfactory. The author is willing to resect 2 diseased parts of the intestinal tract at one operation, but believes that 3 or more anastomoses in series are very rarely justified.

Short-Circuit with Exclusion

This operation has the great advantage that it is performed well away from the inflammatory mass and so is safe. The mortality is low. Some patients have no further trouble. Those that get persistent symptoms or signs, e.g. an external fistula, can have a right hemicolectomy performed very easily 3 months later, when the acute inflammation will have largely subsided. Short-circuit with exclusion is employed when there is a formidable, adherent mass in the right, lower abdomen, or when Crohn's disease is encountered unexpectedly at laparotomy in an obstructed patient who has not been prepared and is not judged to be fit for resection.

A point on the ileum 20 cm proximal to the upper limit of Crohn's disease is selected and the subtending mesentery is carefully divided towards its root for a distance of 5–7 cm. The wall of the ileum is freed from its mesentery for 1 cm on either side of the proposed line of section. Two Schoemaker (or Parker–Kerr) clamps are placed across the ileum, which is divided between them. The distal end is closed and infolded, Fig. 4. First, a continuous 0 chromic catgut stitch (Ethicon, No. 454), loosely circling the clamp blades, is placed. The Schoemaker clamp is withdrawn, and the stitch is pulled tight; the stitch can be brought back along the first suture line to the starting end as a continuous locked stitch. Both ends of the line are then infolded with purse-string stitches of black silk. These are held while a few more silk stitches are inserted between them so as to secure the invagination of the ileal stump.

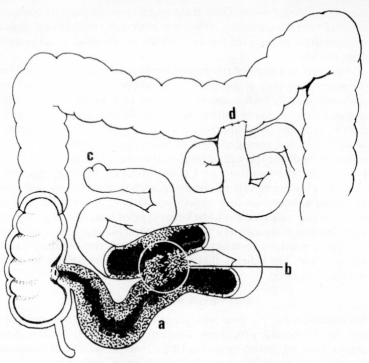

Fig. 4. Short-circuit with exclusion. The diseased ileum (*a*) has been opened
to show the thickened wall and narrow, distorted lumen. There is an
internal fistula (*b*) into an adjacent loop. The ileum has been divided and
closed, (*c*), 20 cm proximal to the diseased segments. Mid-ileum has been
joined end-to-side, (*d*), to the transverse colon.

Depending on the experience of the surgeon and on the diameter of
the proximal ileal opening, either an end-to-side or side-to-side
anastomosis to the middle of the transverse colon can be made. The first
alternative is neater and will be chosen by most experienced operators.
The second type of anastomosis takes a little more time but is safer for
the trainee surgeon. It involves closure of the proximal end, as already
described, and then a lateral anastomosis. For either of these procedures
the middle, dependent part of the transverse colon must be cleared of
fatty encumbrances and be temporarily controlled by an occlusion
clamp. Outer interrupted silk and inner continuous catgut stitches are
used, as for the end-to-end anastomosis after resection (page 172).

It is unwise to attempt to take a biopsy specimen from the diseased
ileum. A short cuff of intestine can be excised between the Schoemaker
clamps and sent to the pathologist to ascertain if it is free from Crohn's
disease.

An accessible enlarged lymph node may also be gently freed and submitted for examination. The peritoneum over it is incised and the node mobilized by blunt dissection. Any small vessels at its poles are seen, caught with Dunhill haemostats, and divided. One of the disadvantages of the short-circuit with exclusion operation is that the glandular and ileal cuff specimens frequently provide no histological confirmation of the diagnosis of Crohn's disease.

"Acute Crohn's Disease"

This may be either an acute presentation or flare-up of genuine Crohn's disease or else some entirely different form of inflammation of the lower ileum. The abdomen has often been opened by a grid-iron incision because appendicitis was suspected. It is likely to be difficult, if not impossible, to make a certain diagnosis. Furthermore, the operator may be inexperienced.

When the ileum is found red and thickened the mesentery should be examined for lymph node enlargement. As much of the small intestine as comes readily is drawn out of the grid-iron incision and is inspected for skip lesions. In a female the right Fallopian tube is examined in case it is the primary site of inflammation.

Complete obstruction is rare and in its absence it is advisable not to interfere any further with the intestine. If the caecal wall is healthy, the appendix is removed and the stump carefully invaginated. Appendicectomy enables acute appendicitis to be excluded from the differential diagnosis should lower abdominal pain recur at a later date (Williams, 1971). The inflamed ileum is returned to the abdomen, which is then closed. Many of these cases are not in fact Crohn's disease, and subsequent investigations fail to reveal any permanent abnormality in the intestine.

Short-circuit with exclusion (through a paramedian incision) is the operation of choice when the patient has gross evidence of obstruction.

Crohn's Disease of Stomach and Duodenum

Chronic granulomatous disease in the gastric antrum and duodenum gives rise to symptoms similar to those of pyloric stenosis. There is almost always disease lower down the alimentary canal. The gastric and duodenal lesions are by-passed by a gastroenterostomy (Burgess *et al.*, 1971). Crohn's disease elsewhere in the abdomen is dealt with on its own merits. Very extensive intestinal resections increase gastric acid output (Fielding *et al.*, 1971), and in theory might cause a stomal ulcer. However, to add a protective vagotomy to the gastroenterostomy might increase steatorrhoea and because of this risk the vagi are mostly left intact.

Treatment of Fistulae

External Fistula
Nearly always there will have been a previous operation. Most fistulae follow drainage of a right iliac fossa abscess or have appeared at variable intervals of time after an exploratory or definitive operation. Copious discharge from the incision within a few days suggests leakage from a suture line. Williams (1971) thinks that many of these leaks heal spontaneously. Not all surgeons take such a sanguine view. With partial breakdown of an anastomosis, the patient's condition can become grave very rapidly. Total parenteral alimentation (page 154) must be started and a broad-spectrum antibiotic given. As soon as the patient can be rendered fit, the abdomen is re-explored, and the old anastomosis repaired or, preferably, a new one fashioned. This kind of disaster is rare.

The common type of single external fistula is not dangerous; it is more of a chronic nuisance because of its intermittent discharge. Multiple fistulae can undermine the patient's health and morale; vigorous pre-operative preparation may be necessary (Enker and Block, 1969).

If it is decided to re-enter the abdomen through the old incision, great care must be exercised because intestine may be stuck to its posterior surface. With an external orifice of a fistula in the right iliac fossa, several Mayo's haemostats are applied to the right edge of the opened parietal peritoneum and are lifted upwards, towards the ceiling. The surgeon may have a better view if he stands on the left of the operating table. The fistulous tract may be a fibrous band, like a pencil, leading from thickened ileum to the anterior abdominal wall; it is easily divided. More often the ileal mass is adherent to the parietes, and the two have to be pinched or prized apart. When this is accomplished, the inner end of the fistula may be seen, but it is suprising how difficult it is to find the tract in some cases. Once mobilized, the ileal mass is resected in the usual manner. The external orifice is often in a grid-iron scar. It is simply curetted and the Sterivac drain may be led out through it. In the few cases where it is considered too hazardous to free the mass, short-circuit with exclusion will often permit the fistula to heal.

When the external fistula is in a paramedian scar, the new incision should surround the orifice. The peritoneum is opened as far away from it as possible and, working from each side in turn, the intestine affected by Crohn's disease is gradually detached from the abdominal wall and resected.

Internal Fistula
Many internal fistulae are only discovered at operation, and by themselves would not appear to have given rise to any additional or more

severe symptoms of Crohn's disease. When the fistula is between two adjacent loops of ileum, or between lower ileum and caecum or ascending colon, all the affected parts can be removed *en bloc*. Intestine which has a fistula entering it should be regarded as being involved in the chronic granulomatous process. When the other end of the fistula opens into the intestine some distance away from the principal site of disease, then a separate segmental resection will be required to remove it. The main exception to this rule is when a fistula is connected to the duodenum. Segments of duodenum cannot be resected. After detaching the fistula, the defect in the duodenum is closed transversely in two layers. There is always a considerable risk of leakage when unhealthy tissues are sutured together. Nevertheless, 3 patients were treated successfully in the above manner at Mount Sinai Hospital (Leichtling and Garlock 1962).

Ileo-vesical Fistula (see page 127).
Ileo-vaginal Fistula (see page 128).

Operations for Recurrent Symptoms

The reappearance of abdominal pain some time after a primary operation may mean: (*a*) adhesions or kinking are causing simple mechanical obstruction; (*b*) reactivation of disease left within the abdomen, e.g. in an excluded loop or skip lesion; (*c*) true recurrence with fresh areas of Crohn's disease developing, mostly in the small bowel just proximal to the site of the first operation.

Adhesions and mechanical distortion at an anastomosis are unlikely to cause serious deterioration in the patient's general health unless there has been prolonged vomiting. The occult blood test on the stool is negative and the ESR and haemoglobin are mostly normal. Symptoms are likely to persist unless another operation is performed.

Before embarking on any second or later operative procedure, it is advisable to read the notes written by the surgeon on the first occasion, and, by barium meal and enema studies, to determine the site of the new abnormality as accurately as possible. By careful dissection the old anastomosis can usually be freed. If adhesions are dense and there is no sign of active inflammation, it is wiser simply to perform a side-to-side anastomosis between the loop of bowel entering and the one that leaves the tethered down zone or encapsulated mass. A fistula is likely to follow over-enthusiastic attempts to unravel loops firmly stuck together.

Reactivation of disease in an excluded loop means that the bypass procedure has failed and the lower, blind loop of ileum should be removed. The ascending colon may be perfectly healthy, in which case the proximal ileum can be detached from the transverse colon and joined to the ascending colon, as in a primary resection and anastomosis; the old stoma in the transverse colon is closed in two layers. In an unfit patient it is quicker to do a right hemicolectomy, dividing and closing the transverse colon to the right of the original anastomosis.

In any second operation it is always worth looking for any unusual arrangement of the intestines which might be restored to normal. In an emergency operation on an obstructed patient, a long length of healthy intestine may inadvertently have been bypassed. This may profitably be reinserted into the intestinal tract.

A skip lesion that has stenosed down to cause sub-acute obstruction may be resected. If multiple skip lesions are noted, only the one or two seen to be narrowing the lumen are short-circuited. Medical treatment is given afterwards for the residual Crohn's disease.

Recurrence of Crohn's disease in a piece of intestine previously un-affected does not necessarily give rise to disabling symptoms. Many patients have only occasional colic and a slight increase in their diarrhoea. They respond to drug therapy and are often able to continue working. Further operative intervention should only be contemplated (i) when there are compelling mechanical reasons for same, and the disease is well localized; (ii) for the small number of cases that derive no benefit from medical treatment, and whose general health is deteri-orating. Rapid return of symptoms after operation suggests that the disease is widespread, and consequently that further surgery has little to offer. There are some centres where a policy of salvage surgery is adopted; between 5–20 per cent of all patients attending with Crohn's disease may have had 4 or more abdominal operations (Williams, 1971). A patient should only be subjected to repeated operations for the clearest of reasons and after all the alternatives have been fully explored.

Plenty of time should always be allowed on any operation list for a case of salvage surgery. It often comes as a pleasant surprise in Crohn's disease to find that re-resection is comparatively easy. Again, the intestine is divided about 20 cm proximal to the upper edge of the thickened area, and at a point 4–5 cm beyond its lower limit. The mucosa in the opened ends is inspected before they are sutured together in 2 layers. Thereafter the patient may go for some years without further symptoms. A second recurrence is not very common.

Crohn's Disease of the Colon

The therapeutic approach to colonic Crohn's disease is rather more conservative than when the disease is confined to the small intestine. Thirteen out of 35 Aberdeen patients (37 per cent) with transmural colitis were still being treated medically in mid-1971, at least 18 months after the onset of their symptoms. There are several reasons for per-sisting with medical treatment for a considerable time. The patients on average are older than those with ileal disease; respiratory, cardio-vascular or other degenerative conditions may make them poor risks for general anaesthesia and major surgery. There is a clinical impression —at present it is no more than this—that the medium-term response to drug therapy is reasonably satisfactory. At any rate, the progression or regression of their colonic lesion can be measured with some accuracy by barium enema examinations. Changes can take place very rapidly (Cole and Kyle, 1968). A few patients with complications do have to be operated on urgently. Obstruction is a constant danger with ileal disease, but the much greater diameter of the colon renders obstruction less likely when that part of the intestine alone is involved.

Surgery should not be delayed when carcinoma cannot rapidly be excluded in a patient with one stenotic lesion. There are some types of colitis, with pain, diarrhoea and rectal bleeding, which settle spontaneously within a few weeks. These include ischaemic colitis and evanescent colitis (Miller *et al.*, 1971). Clearly, it would be unwise to perform radical surgery at an early stage in these conditions.

Segmental Resection

If a colonic neoplasm is suspected or a tight simple stricture is seen, the safest course is to excise the lesion, along with a generous margin of normal colon on either side and a wedge of mesentery. When a report of Crohn's disease is received back from the pathologist there is no need for further operation at that time. Further lesions may arise at a later date; if they do, the diagnosis is known and they can be dealt with by whatever method seems appropriate. In older patients there is little place for pre-emptive resection.

Right hemicolectomy has already been mentioned as an extension of ileal resection (page 159). It is a special type of segmental resection, more frequently successful than other local resections for Crohn's disease of the colon. If recurrence takes place years later it is more likely to be on the ileal side of the anastomosis, but it can develop elsewhere in the colon. Excision of the sigmoid loop is worthwhile when it is grossly involved by contact spread from the ileum.

Except in the above circumstances, segmental resection is not generally favoured in Crohn's disease of the colon.

Sub-total Colectomy

Because there are mostly several parts of the colon affected by Crohn's disease ("discontinuous pathology"), when operation is deemed the correct form of treatment a subtotal or total colectomy is practised. The state of the rectum is of vital importance. Surface appearances on sigmoidoscopy are not enough; rectal biopsy specimens have to be examined for evidence of any sub-mucosal oedema or cellular infiltrate. When the rectum is completely normal it is possible to remove the entire colon round to the upper rectum, to which healthy ileum is anastomosed.

The results have not been good, and the recurrence rate has been high. Faulty selection of cases may be partly to blame for these failures.

At Oxford, when there are several areas of Crohn's disease in the colon, but both caecum and rectum are healthy, the operation shown in Figs. 5 and 6 has been tried (Webster, 1971). The colon is divided at

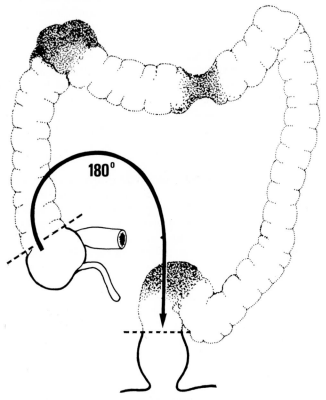

FIG. 5. The Oxford operation for Crohn's disease of the colon. When caecum and rectum are normal, they are joined by rotating the caecum through 180° after performing a sub-total colectomy.

the upper borders of caecum and of rectum, and is removed. The caecum is then rotated to the left through 180° and anastomosed end-to-end in 2 layers to the top of the rectum. A Foley catheter, brought out through the appendix stump, provides temporary decompression. The advantage of this operation is that although the water-absorbing colonic mucosa has been lost, the ileo-caecal valve is preserved. The state of the rectum and the anastomosis can be ascertained by performing a sigmoidoscopy.

An occasional patient with a normal rectum has ano-rectal infection and fistulae. There is a chance that these lesions will heal on being treated by conventional surgical techniques, e.g. drainage of abscess, fistulectomy, once the disease higher up in the colon has been removed (Goligher, 1967).

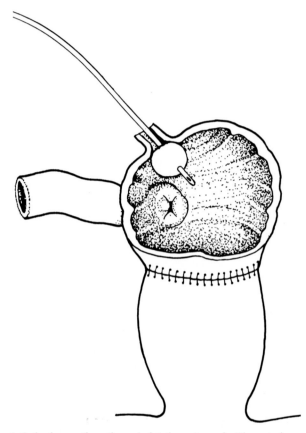

Fig. 6. Oxford operation: the completed anastomosis. The anterior wall of the caecum has been cut away to show the ileo-caecal valve and the small Foley catheter brought out through the appendix stump.

Proctocolectomy

With Crohn's disease widely scattered throughout colon and rectum, and frequently present in the terminal ileum as well, proctocolectomy with ileostomy is the treatment of choice. Out of an operative series of 62 patients, Goligher (1967) treated 33 (53 per cent) by this method. He has removed up to 180 cm of ileum in continuity with the colon and still had a manageable ileostomy. When there are numerous perianal fistulae associated with diseased colon and rectum, proctocolectomy should be carried out if and when the patient is fit (Cole *et al.*, 1969).

The operation is performed with the patient in the Lloyd-Davies (1939) position, as for a synchronous combined excision of rectum. Wide excision of perianal skin may be necessary in order to remove all the fistulae, but apart from this the operators keep close to the rectal wall, away from the nervi erigentes and ureters. The ileostomy may be brought out extra-peritoneally (Goligher, 1967) at a pre-selected site in the right iliac fossa, or the cut edge of the mesentery may be hitched to the anterior and lateral abdominal wall (Brooke, 1954). The ileostomy itself is of the everted, mucosa-to-skin type that is standard for ulcerative colitic patients. A disposable ileostomy bag (Chiron or Hollister, with karaya gum seal) is applied before the patient leaves the theatre.

The edges of the levator ani muscles and fatty tissues in the perineum are approximated with interrupted catgut stitches. The perineal wound is drained. A major disappointment in this operation has been the delay in healing of the perineum. Nearly half the wounds may not be completely healed after 12 months (Ritchie, 1971). Zinc sulphate, 110 mg per day, may be tried to see if it will aid the reparative process.

An operation to fashion an intra-abdominal reservoir from a U-loop of ileum, and thereby to enable the patient to dispense with an external ileostomy appliance, has been developed in Göteborg (Kock, 1971); it is still being evaluated.

Other Operations

Diversion procedures, with the hope of resting inflamed bowel and eventually being able to restore its continuity, have been tried in Crohn's disease of the colon (or rarely, of ileum). Truelove *et al.* (1965) at Oxford described a double-barrelled ileostomy technique. In California, Kivel *et al.* (1967) brought out the proximal end as a standard ileostomy on the right side, and the distal ileum, on the left side, as a mucous fistula. Their 21 patients appear to have had moderately severe colonic disease, with a mean weight loss of 29 lb (13 kg). Biopsy specimens were taken from diseased colon and lymph nodes. The early results were good in all cases. However, 7 patients (33 per cent) suffered a recrudescence of their disease between 5 and 36 months after their first operation and they finally required proctocolectomy. Eight patients remained asymptomatic. In only 6 patients was restoration of continuity attempted, after challenging the colonic mucosa with injected ileostomy contents for some weeks. Three out of the 6 patients developed recurrent symptoms within a few months (Oberhelman and Kohatsu, 1971), and as a result enthusiasm for this mode of therapy has become somewhat dampened. A trial of intestinal diversion was carried out in

Birmingham (Burman *et al.*, 1971), and Williams (1971) now doubts whether defunctioned bowel can be successfully used again.

One Aberdeen patient had Crohn's disease in rectum, sigmoid and descending colon. He refused to have his rectum taken out, so a left hemicolectomy, with permanent transverse colostomy, was performed 5 years ago. There has been no proximal extension of his disease. However, although no longer exposed to the faecal stream, his rectal disease has not subsided and biopsy specimens reveal significant inflammatory changes. Considering the pathology of Crohn's disease, it does seem unlikely that intestine which has been the site of active transmural inflammation for many months or years will ever be capable of reverting to complete normality.

References

Barker, K., Graham, N. G., Mason, M. C., de Dombal, F. T. and Goligher, J. C. (1971), *Brit. J. Surg.*, **58**, 270.

Brooke, B. N. (1954), *Ulcerative Colitis and its Surgical Treatment*. Edinburgh: Livingstone.

Burgess, J. N., Legge, D. A. and Judd, E. S. (1971), *Surg. Gynec. Obstet.*, **132**, 628.

Burman, J. H., Cooke, W. T. and Williams, J. A. (1971), *Gut*, **12**, 432.

Burman, J. H., Thompson, H., Cooke, W. T. and Williams, J. A. (1971), *Gut*, **12**, 11.

Cole, T. P. and Kyle, J. (1968), *Bull. Int. Soc. Chir.*, **27**, 402.

Cole, T. P., Ewen, S. W. B. and Kyle, J. (1969), in *Progress in Proctology*. Ed. J. Hoferichter, p. 44. Berlin: Springer Verlag.

Crohn, B. B. (1957), *Arch. Surg. (Chicago)*, **74**, 305.

de Dombal, F. T., Burton, I. and Goligher, J. C. (1971), *Brit. J. Surg.*, **58**, 805.

Enker, W. E. and Block, G. E. (1969), *Arch. Surg. (Chicago)*, **98**, 493.

Fielding, J. F., Cooke, W. T. and Williams, J. A. (1971), *Lancet*, **1**, 1106.

Garlock, J. H. (1967), *Surgery of the Alimentary Tract*, p. 241. New York: Appleton–Century–Crofts.

Goligher, J. C. (1967), *Surgery of the Anus, Rectum and Colon*, p. 974. London: Bailliere, Tindall & Cassell.

Kivel, R. M., Taylor, K. B. and Oberhelman, H. (1967), *Lancet*, **2**, 632.

Kock, N. G. (1971), *Ann. Surg.*, **173**, 545.

Krause, U. (1971), *Scand. J. Surg.*, **6**, 479.

Kyle, J. (1964), *Austral. N.Z. J. Surg.*, **34**, 116.

Leichtling, J. J. and Garlock, J. H. (1962), *Gastroenterology*, **43**, 151.

Lloyd-Davies, O. V. (1939), *Lancet*, **2**, 74.

Miller, W. T., De Poto, D. W., Scholl, H. W. and Raffensperger, E. C. (1971), *Radiology*, **100**, 71.

Morson, B. C. (1971), *Scand. J. Gastroent.*, **6**, 573.

Oberhelman, H. A. and Kohatsu, S. (1971), in *Regional Enteritis (Crohn's Disease)*. Ed. A. Engel and T. Larsson, p. 195. Stockholm: Skandia International Symposia.

Ritchie, J. K. (1971), *Gut*, **12**, 528.

Truelove, S. C., Ellis, H. and Webster, C. U. (1965), *Brit. med. J.*, **1**, 150.

Wallensten, S. (1971), in *Regional Enteritis (Crohn's Disease)*. Ed. A. Engel and T. Larsson, p. 192. Stockholm: Skandia International Symposia.

Weakley, F. L. and Turnbull, R. B. (1971), *Dis. Col. Rectum*, **14**, 17.

Webster, C. U. (1971), Roy. Coll. Surg. Edin. Meeting, 18th October, 1971.

Wenckert, A., Brahme, F. and Nilssen, T. (1971), *Nord. Med.*, **83**, 334.

Williams, J. A. (1971), *Gut*, **12**, 739.

Chapter X
Prognosis

It is very difficult to foretell what the future holds for any person who develops Crohn's disease. In general, the behaviour of the disease is unpredictable and may vary very markedly between one patient and another. When disease activity is presumably low and symptoms slight, a patient may wait many years before attending hospital for the special investigations or laparotomy necessary to establish the diagnosis. At the other extreme, a previously healthy person may have to be operated on within hours of the onset of symptoms, because of suspected appendicitis.

The history obtained at the time of making the diagnosis is of little assistance in predicting what will happen thereafter. Only one thing is certain: if the diagnosis of chronic Crohn's disease is correct, then the condition will not vanish spontaneously and permanently. The course that the disease may follow is infinitely variable. At the one extreme a patient may go progressively downhill and die within a few weeks in spite of radical surgery and every available supportive measure. At the other end of the spectrum, a patient may survive for many years, without radical resection, and in tolerably good health. The best known example of the latter, fortunate type of patient, was the 34th President of the United States of America, Dwight D. Eisenhower. He lived for 46 years after the onset of Crohn's disease (Heaton, 1964; Hughes *et al.*, 1971), and held the highest offices in the land in both peace and war. For the majority of patients, the disease will pursue its erratic course somewhere between these two extremes. There will be exacerbations of inflammation, therapeutic hazards to be circumvented and surgical vicissitudes to be overcome. However, it would be rather misleading to describe these events as punctuating the course of disease that has not been extirpated. It is more accurate to regard them as superimposed on a background of sub-optimal health in most patients.

With its aetiology still a mystery, there is no specific cure for Crohn's disease. Some of the therapeutic measures used are of doubtful efficacy, or if they are in some measure beneficial, this effect may only become apparent after a considerable time. Consequently changes of treatment are the rule rather than the exception, even though any one line of treatment may be pursued for many months. Some operations that have been practised are useless and do nothing more than mark the start of what eventually becomes a long series of increasingly radical procedures.

Because the factors affecting the inflammatory process in the intestine are not understood and the weapons available for controlling it are not very effective, few workers have attempted to give an overall picture of the prognosis in Crohn's disease. The numbers of possible permutations and combinations between the natural progression of the disease and varying therapeutic efforts are very large indeed. The best attempt to demonstrate the possible outcomes is that contained in the final part of the Mayo Clinic report (van Patter *et al.*, 1954). By its very complexity—by the multiplicity of its tables, the addition of operations for some patients, the subtraction of patients from other groups—this report epitomizes the difficulties that confront a doctor when he is trying to give an honest prognosis to a patient who has Crohn's disease.

It is an over-simplification, but it does make interpretation easier, if prognosis is considered under four main headings: (1) untreated patients; (2) non-operative therapy; (3) results of different surgical procedures; (4) overall mortality. Knowing what the various therapeutic options have to offer and that the intrinsic nature of the disease is the most important factor, the doctor can make a guarded statement to his patient about the future. Because it offers the best prospect of long periods of good health, ileal resection is considered in some detail.

Untreated Patients

Spontaneous disappearance of proven, chronic Crohn's disease has not been reported. However, this simple statement does require some qualification. It may be very difficult to "prove" that a patient really had Crohn's disease without histological confirmation of the diagnosis. Understanding of the clinical features and radiological appearances has steadily improved over the last four decades, so that the degree of certainty about the diagnosis has increased. Nevertheless, some experienced clinicians would contend that the alleged spontaneous cure of what was thought to be Crohn's disease would in itself be enough to refute all evidence except that obtained from the final arbiter of diagnostic problems, the microscope.

Among the 600 patients seen at the Mayo Clinic in the years (before steroids) up to 1950, there were 26 for whom surgery was advised but who refused treatment. It was possible to follow up 20 of these patients. Eleven had eventually been forced to have operations elsewhere, 6 (30 per cent) had died as a result of their Crohn's disease, 2 were described as "ill", only one was in fair condition, and no patient was described as being well. This small group of patients demonstrates what is liable to happen if one of the more potent remedies, such as corticosteroids, immunosuppressive drugs or radical resection, is not employed.

Medical Therapy

Several decades ago about 90 per cent of patients with Crohn's disease eventually required an operation (Crohn and Yarnis, 1958; Colcock and Vansant, 1960; Davis, 1961). Medical therapy before 1950 was directed towards the relief of symptoms and replacing deficiencies of iron, vitamins and other essential substances. It would be wrong to think that the results obtained with these simple measures represent those that might be achieved in the future with broad-spectrum antibiotics, corticosteroids and immunosuppressive agents. The drugs that have become available during the last two decades can probably modify the inflammatory process, even though they are unable to prevent or to cure it. None has been submitted to a prolonged, double-blind, prospective trial on a large scale. At the present time it is not known if they arrest or reverse the inflammation in some lesions. The dangers of prolonged use of antibiotics are well known. Resistant strains of bacteria are produced and there may be a serious overgrowth of fungi.

Corticosteroids (or corticotrophin) need to be given in adequate dosage, equivalent to at least 100 mg of cortisone per day. In a series of 105 patients with Crohn's disease at the Central Middlesex Hospital, London, Jones and Lennard-Jones (1967) reported that initially 30 patients were given steroids. Only 3 patients (10 per cent) went into remission, that is they remained free from symptoms 6 months after stopping treatment. Sixty-three per cent were temporarily improved but soon relapsed when steroids were discontinued; further medical treatment or resection had to be undertaken. Six out of the 30 steroid-treated patients (20 per cent) eventually died. The addition of anti-tuberculous drugs made no difference to the results. Sparberg and Kirsner (1966) agreed that the response to steroids was variable and unpredictable. To them it appeared that steroid therapy was most likely to succeed in young patients, with short histories, who had not had any previous operations. Complications attributable to long-term steroid administration did occur, but were reversible. Other workers have considered the possibility that there may be some relationship between corticosteroid therapy and the later development of malignant hypertension (Prior et al., 1970) and perforation and fistula formation (Jones and Lennard-Jones, 1966; Brill et al., 1969). No serious complications of steroid therapy have been seen in the Aberdeen patients. Nevertheless, many doctors view the long-term use of steroids with considerable disquiet (Goldstein et al., 1967). The risks inherent in their use do not appear excessive for, and may have to be accepted by, patients with very extensive or recurrent disease causing malabsorptive defects (Gump and Lepore, 1960).

Immunosuppressive agents in high dosage are always liable to produce such severe bone marrow depression that uncontrollable infection develops and kills the patient. There is considerable variation in patient tolerance to these drugs (Patterson *et al.*, 1971). In addition there may be some risk of their producing lymphomatous tumours when given for long periods (Doak *et al.*, 1968).

In spite of these hazards and the uncertain response, medical measures have in the recent past been used in more patients with Crohn's disease and have been employed for much longer periods of time than was once the case. At the beginning of 1968, in Aberdeen, out of a total of 145 patients, approximately 25 per cent had received medical treatment alone. The results certainly were not good; 3 patients died and less than half the survivors were well. Medical treatment here means at least one month of the type of combined therapy outlined in Chapter VIII; in earlier years it had failed in 45 cases. Some minor operations, such as a laparotomy or drainage, have been disregarded in these figures for medical treatment. Almost inexorably patients seemed to progress towards resection. By the end of the 1960's, the "medical salvage rate" for the Aberdeen Series was 11 per cent; this rate corresponds closely with the 10·3 per cent from the Presbyterian Hospital, New York (Gump and Lepore, 1960). Three years later, more patients are being submitted to resection, mostly after an intensive course of medical treatment has brought about an improvement in their general condition, and local inflammation has been reduced in its intensity.

More than 30 per cent of those Aberdeen patients who have Crohn's disease of the colon have been satisfactorily controlled by non-operative measures; Yarnis and Crohn (1960) had obtained a good response to steroid therapy in this type of patient. Other workers (Lewin and Swales, 1966; Slaney, 1968) consider that colonic cases do badly on medical treatment. Marshak *et al.* (1966) believe that medical measures should be persisted with so long as the patient shows no evidence of deterioration. Eventually, about 70 per cent of cases may require major surgery (Korelitz, 1967). The potential late danger in medical treatment for colonic Crohn's disease is the development of carcinoma in the colon. The size of this risk is not known in 1972. In the patients with colonic and rectal disease studied by Brill *et al.* (1969) carcinoma supervened in 7·4 per cent, while Lewin and Swales (1966) reported an incidence of 15 per cent. Young patients can be affected (Kipping, 1970).

Prognosis after Operation

By a combination of medical and surgical treatment, 4 out of 5 patients with Crohn's disease can be restored to full activity (Stahlgren and Ferguson, 1961). A variety of complications may follow operation (Goldstein *et al.*, 1968) but even after radical resection the nutritional status of the patient is mostly good (Wallensten, 1971). The possible late appearance of gall-stones has been considered on page 134.

Patients are more likely to experience long-lasting relief of symptoms after surgery than after medical treatment (Burton *et al.*, 1969). The operations that may be performed in Crohn's disease fall into three groups from the point of view of prognosis—

   (1) Diagnostic Exploration—this group would include patients who had appendicectomies, but exclude all cases where an attempt at eradication of the disease had been made. The prognosis will be that of surgically untreated disease.

   (2) Emergency Procedures—most of this group would consist of patients in whom a simple short-circuit had been performed because of acute obstruction, adhesions or other circumstances that made more radical procedures inadvisable. Before 1950 a simple diversion procedure was often carried out in the hope that it might cure the patient.

   (3) Definitive Operations—these may be either short-circuiting with exclusion, so removing the diseased bowel from the faecal stream, or else radical resection where, at the end of the operation, all visible diseased bowel has been removed from the abdomen.

The candidate for surgery will be interested, first, in his chances of surviving the operation and, second, in the prospects of being permanently free of Crohn's disease.

Operative Mortality

Death within 28 days of operation for Crohn's disease should now be rare. There is a slight risk attached to any laparotomy, and some patients will be malnourished. Emergency operations always carry a higher mortality than elective procedures; with acute obstruction it may be 5–10 per cent, and when perforation has occurred the mortality is likely to be 25–30 per cent. The toll of deaths inseparable from emergency operations is a strong argument in favour of earlier elective operations.

For short-circuit with exclusion the operative mortality varies from 1 per cent (van Patter *et al.*, 1954) to 5 per cent (Atwell *et al.*, 1965); some of the deaths in the more recent series may have been the result of performing this type of diversion in emergency circumstances. There were no deaths in the 21 patients in the Aberdeen series on whom it was performed electively.

For the 265 patients who had primary resections at the Mayo Clinic the operative mortality was 2·3 per cent; there were no deaths in the last 100 cases. Although many of their patients were emaciated, there was no mortality in the Calcutta series (Gupta *et al.*, 1962). One of the 62 Aberdeen patients died following primary resection for Crohn's disease of the ileum. Crismer and Dreze (1962) had a resection mortality of 1·9 per cent in Liege. At Leeds, de Dombal *et al.* (1971) noted that the early mortality in patients aged over 50 years was 4 times that in younger patients. Second and subsequent operations carried a mortality double (8·2 per cent) that of primary procedures (4·1 per cent). In this

Leeds series, accumulated over many years, approximately 1 patient out of every 3 sooner or later required a further operation. When second and later operations are required, the technical difficulties within the abdomen will be greater and generally the patient's condition will be poor, so that inevitably there is an increased mortality. The operative mortality tended to be higher with colonic disease, probably on account of the more extensive nature of the operation, and the need for urgent surgery in some of these cases.

Operative Morbidity

Following definitive surgery approximately 25 per cent of patients develop postoperative complications, mainly wound sepsis and fistulae (Latchis *et al.*, 1971).

Late Results

Although a tendency to recur is unfortunately a feature of Crohn's disease, almost 90 per cent of patients express themselves as being satisfied with the result of operation. Good health is enjoyed for 72 per cent of patient-years; weight is gained and the chief symptoms are relieved in most cases (de Dombal *et al.*, 1971).

Recurrence

Davis (1961) has drawn attention to the difference between *reactivation* of the inflammatory process in previously unhealthy intestine, and the appearance after operation of granulomatous disease in a part of the intestinal tract that had previously looked normal. It is in this latter sense that the term *recurrence* is used here. A few patients can have radiological or other evidence of recurrent disease and yet have no symptoms referable to it. Van Patter *et al.* (1954) also had difficulty in defining recurrence. They were more certain of the converse state, arrest of the disease—"no reappearance in structures carrying the main faecal stream after 2 years". They knew that Crohn's disease could reappear, and kill, many years after what had been considered to be a curative operation on the small intestine.

By definition, acute Crohn's disease does not recur; all signs and symptoms will have permanently disappeared within 4 weeks of the onset. After laparotomy for chronic Crohn's disease further symptoms are to be expected. In Aberdeen 43 patients began by having a laparotomy; by early 1968 only 9 (20 per cent) were still free of major symptoms, while 4 had had diversion with exclusion procedures and 18 had progressed to resection. Two of the patients had died at home from intestinal obstruction, presumably as a result of Crohn's disease.

Recurrence takes place very quickly after simple short-circuit. In the Mayo Clinic series, the disease was arrested in only 12 patients out of

100 having this type of operation. Fistulae did not heal and most patients soon needed further surgery. The experience at Leeds (Atwell *et al.*, 1965) has been similar.

When the diseased intestine is excluded from the faecal stream, the results are rather better. In 1968, out of 26 patients (including emergencies) who had had short-circuit with exclusion operations in Aberdeen, 7 (28 per cent) were well; 5 had died some years after their operation. At the Mayo Clinic approximately 40 per cent were arrested by diversion with exclusion, but 55 per cent developed recurrences. Only one excluded ileal loop in the Aberdeen series had to be resected because of the onset of megaloblastic anaemia. However, Garlock and Crohn (1945) were forced to excise 27 per cent of excluded, diseased loops on account of troublesome symptoms.

Crohn's Disease of the Colon

Having only been widely recognized for the past decade, Crohn's disease of the colon has not been followed up for as long as the ileal form of the disease. It may affect a slightly different age group and respond differently to treatment. The results of operation in the two types of disease are therefore considered separately, but only those for ileal disease are dealt with in detail and prognostic factors evaluated.

Thirteen out of the 35 patients seen in Aberdeen with Crohn's disease of colon and rectum did not have any major operation, although several of them had positive rectal biopsies; 3 of them had fistulectomies or abscesses drained. Twenty-two patients had definitive resections, 3 being proctocolectomies with terminal ileostomies; 2 patients had ileo-rectal anastomoses. One elderly female died 4 weeks after an abdomino-perineal excision of rectum and left colon. The follow-up period is short, varying from 1 to 6 years. Seventeen patients (77 per cent) are well, and only 4 are still having symptoms. The ileostomies in the Aberdeen patients have not given any trouble; in Cleveland, 20 per cent developed ileitis proximal to the stoma (Farmer *et al.*, 1968). Some Leeds patients had minor skin irritations (de Dombal *et al.*, 1971b). Ileo-rectal anastomoses are less satisfactory (Burman *et al.*, 1970): leaks occurred in 32 per cent of a series of 25 patients who had continuity re-established by this method; 3 patients died and 15 (60 per cent) developed recurrent disease.

Cornes and Strecher (1961) believed that the prognosis of Crohn's disease of the colon was much better than that of Crohn's lesions of the small intestine. de Dombal *et al.* (1971b) share this view, 96 per cent of their surviving colonic cases being in good or excellent health at the time of follow-up. If Crohn's disease continues to appear in the colon and rectum of elderly people, then their advanced age will itself become a major factor in prognosis. However, recurrence is less likely in old people with colonic disease (de Dombal *et al.*, 1971a). The outlook may be worst in patients with combined disease of ileum and colon (Kent *et al.*, 1970).

Resection for Ileal Disease

Because 80 per cent of patients have Crohn's disease affecting the ileum alone or along with the adjacent caecum, whatever line of treatment is found most satisfactory for this type of disease will confer benefit on the greatest number of patients. It is therefore worthwhile studying the long-term results of resection in some detail, and attempting to analyse factors that may influence the outcome.

Unfortunately recurrence and mortality figures produced by surgeons in the past cannot be used for meaningful comparisons. The duration of follow-up has varied (or not been stated) in different series, and frequently no definition has been given of what has been called a recurrence. The results for all types of surgical procedures have been taken together. The only definitive results for ileal resection that are suitable for comparison are those reported by Lennard-Jones and Stalder (1967).

These workers collected 73 patients who had had first resections for ileal disease at the Central Middlesex Hospital and St. Mark's Hospital, London, between 1949 and 1967. Nine of the patients from this London series had previously had unsuccessful short-circuiting procedures. Two died immediately following resection, leaving 71 patients for follow-up study. The results were analysed by constructing life tables (Hill, 1966). For each of the 10 years following operation the number of patients at risk at the start of the year was calculated; the number of recurrences each year was known, so allowing the proportion developing a recurrence to be accurately determined. Patients dying were subtracted from the total at risk and, by convention, patients followed for only part of a year were reckoned as having been followed for half a year.

The definition of symptomatic recurrence which Lennard-Jones and Stalder adopted was an increase in diarrhoea associated with a return of abdominal pain and loss of weight. They appreciated that after ileal resection or right hemicolectomy a patient's bowels will probably open 2–4 times per 24 hours. It was only when frequency increased at the same time as other symptoms of Crohn's disease reappeared that they considered that recurrence had taken place. The definition may slightly over-estimate the recurrence rate because stenosis at an otherwise healthy anastomosis might produce similar symptoms. Nevertheless, it is these symptoms that the patient is likely to use in judging the success or failure of his operation; they will determine the quality of the life he leads.

In the Aberdeen series up to the end of 1967, there were 62 patients who had undergone primary ileal resection for chronic Crohn's disease (Kyle, 1971). Eight had previously had diversion procedures, 18 had had laparotomies, one had had a nephrectomy for an obstructed ureter and one patient had had a free perforation of Crohn's disease oversewn—in other words, many patients obviously had a relatively severe form of Crohn's disease. The diagnosis was confirmed histologically in all cases. Apart from those who died, no patient was lost to follow-up for 5 years among the pre-1965 group; all the 1965–1967 patients were followed until the end of 1969. The results, calculated in the same manner as those of Lennard-Jones and Stalder (1967), are given in Table 1.

In the years up to the 5th anniversary of their resection, approximately 20 per cent of patients had developed a symptomatic recurrence; by the 10th year 33 per cent had recurrences. The corresponding figures for the London series of patients are 31 per cent and 58 per cent respectively; it must be remembered that these patients were operated on some 6–8 years earlier than those in Aberdeen. Table 1 also confirms

Table 1

*Patients developing a recurrence of symptoms in each of the first
10 years after a first resection for ileal disease*

Year after operation	Well at beginning of year	Lost to follow-up during year	Well, observed only part of year	Exposed to risk of relapse	Number of relapses	Proportion with relapse	Proportion without relapse	Estimated proportion Without relapse to end each year	With relapse to end each year
0	61	0	0	61	6	0·098	0·902	0·902	0·098
1	55	1	0	54·5	2	0·037	0·963	0·869	0·131
2	52	0	0	52	2	0·038	0·962	0·836	0·164
3	50	0	5	47·5	1	0·021	0·979	0·818	0·182
4	44	0	4	42	0	0·000	1·000	0·818	0·182
5	40	1	2	38·5	1	0·026	0·974	0·797	0·203
6	36	0	7	32·5	2	0·062	0·938	0·747	0·253
7	27	0	4	25	0	0·000	1·000	0·747	0·253
8	23	0	3	21·5	1	0·047	0·953	0·712	0·288
9	19	0	7	15·5	1	0·065	0·935	0·666	0·334

the statement of Crohn and Yarnis (1958) that recurrence usually takes place within the first three years after operation. Some patients with recurrent disease are in relatively good health (Kiefer, 1955; de Dombal *et al.*, 1971a), and respond to medical treatment.

Stricter criteria for recurrence have been used, such as radiological deformity and necessity for further resection; they have not been applied to the Aberdeen patients. Postoperative radiological appearances are very difficult to interpret. Surgeons may complain that few radiologists ever come into the operating theatre to see the very oblique or other bizarre anastomoses that they may have to fashion in Crohn's disease. Conversely, radiologists can justifiably complain that few details about previous operations may be given to them on request forms for repeat barium examinations. When Lennard-Jones and Stalder applied the stricter criteria mentioned above to their data from London, they reduced both the 5 year and 10 year recurrence rates by about 7·5 per cent.

The chances of recurrence after a second resection may be greater than after a primary excision of ileum (van Patter *et al.*, 1954) or be unaffected by previous operations (de Dombal *et al.*, 1971). In the London series, the calculated probability of recurrence after a second resection was about twice as great as after the first operation. If a programme of re-resection is followed, the patient may finally be left with very little small intestine. Nutrition becomes permanently impaired if more than 60 per cent has been excised (Chen, 1969). Very extensive resections of small intestine, leaving only 60–120 cm in position, make it almost impossible to maintain adequate nutrition; gastric hypersecretion (Windsor *et al.*, 1969) and even sub-acute combined degeneration of the spinal cord may develop (Best, 1959). These sequelae have not been seen in Aberdeen. At the Lahey Clinic 6·8 per cent of patients were left with a short-bowel syndrome (Latchis *et al.*, 1971).

Factors Influencing Recurrence

Age of Onset. Stahlgern and Ferguson (1961) believed that recurrence was more likely when Crohn's disease started in early adult life; Atwell *et al.* (1964) thought the prognosis particularly bad when the onset was before the age of 15 years. However, Lennard-Jones and Stalder divided their patients into 2 approximately equal groups above and below the age of 35 years; the probability of recurrence was identical for the 2 groups. Thirty years of age was found more suitable for dividing the Aberdeen series and the results are given in Table 2. There is a suggestion that patients whose disease started in the first 3 decades of life fare rather worse than older people. However, old patients are by no means immune from recurrence (Gump and Lepore, 1960).

Sex. Table 2 also demonstrates the effect of sex on the chances of

Table 2
Effect of age and sex on estimated proportion of patients with a recurrence within 5 years of first ileal resection in Aberdeen

Factors analyzed	No. in group*	Proportion with recurrence
Age: Under 30 years	32	0·22
30 years and over	29	0·14
Sex: Male (mean age 29 years)	23	0·13
Female (mean age 33 years)	38	0·21
Age/Sex: Under 30 years, male	13	0·08
Under 30 years, female	19	0·32
30 years and over, male	10	0·20
30 years and over, female	19	0·11

* Total of 61 excludes one operative death.

developing a recurrence. Females had the poorer prospect. In the Aberdeen series of resections 62 per cent of the patients were females, compared to only 41 per cent in Lennard-Jones and Stalder's patients. In the latter series the proportion of males in whom recurrence appeared was only slightly less than that for females.

When age at onset and sex are considered together there does seem to be a tendency for younger females not to have such a good prognosis as males of corresponding age. However, all these estimations are based on small numbers and should be interpreted with caution.

Duration of Symptoms. The importance of sub-dividing results at the correct point in order to make comparisons is clearly illustrated in Table 3. When patients who had had symptoms for less than 2 years

Table 3
Influence of the duration of symptoms before ideal resection on the proportion of patients developing recurrent Crohn's disease within 5 years

Pre-operative duration		No. in group*	Proportion with recurrence
Duration only:	Under 2 years	46	0·14
	2 years and over	14	0·20
Duration/Sex:	6 months and less, male	12	0·08
	6 months and less, female	19	0·32
	Over 6 months, male	10	0·20
	Over 6 months, female	19	0·11

* Total of 60 excludes one operative and one accidental death.

were compared with those having longer histories, it appeared that the latter group did worse as regards recurrence. Two years was the dividing point used by Lennard-Jones and Stalder (1967), and it was close to the mean duration of symptoms prior to operation (1·9 years) in the Aberdeen series. However, the proportions relapsing look different when 6 months is chosen (the median duration was 0·8 years) and the sexes considered separately. Females with a short history did worse than other groups, but the numbers are very small. The risk of recurrence was greater among the Leeds patients when symptoms had been present for only a short time (de Dombal *et al.*, 1971a).

Erythrocyte Sedimentation Rate. In 31 out of the 40 patients who never relapsed after resection the mean pre-operative ESR was 30 mm/hr (range: 4–87 mm/hr). For 13 out of the 20 patients in whom Crohn's disease eventually reappeared the mean value was 39 mm/hr (range: 5–102 mm/hr). The patients in whom no ESR was recorded before resection were in the earlier part of the Aberdeen series. The ESR is of no prognostic value. Changes in gamma globulins have been found useful in severe attacks of ulcerative colitis (de Dombal, 1968), while α_2 globulins are often raised in Crohn's disease (Atwell *et al.*, 1965). Prolonged studies will be necessary to determine whether these globulins, the seromucoids or immunoglobulin levels are of prognostic significance. Gross steatorrhoea before operation probably indicates that there is widespread mucosal involvement (Cooke, 1955) and the chances of success following resection must be regarded as slim.

Medical Therapy. In patients who had had a lengthy trial of medical treatment before coming to resection, Gump and Lepore (1960) found that up to 10 years afterwards the results were similar to those noted in patients who had had a resection at an early stage in their illness. It might have been expected that those patients who could have been managed for many months or years on medical therapy would have done well after resection. The forms of medical therapy available 20–30 years ago were different from those that are in use today. The effects of earlier medical treatment on the outcome of resection have not been studied in the Aberdeen or London series.

There is a need for controlled trials of the effects of drugs such as sulphasalazine and azathioprine on the incidence of recurrent disease after resection. Corticosteroids seem to have no effect, but there has been no blind, prospective study. One of the reasons for advocating surgery is to avoid the necessity of constantly having to take drugs.

Findings at Operation. It is unfortunate that many operation notes lack details that would be of interest from the point of view of prognosis. For example, it is frequently not clear whether lymph nodes in the mesentery were pathologically enlarged, or were simply more obvious than usual in the thin mesentery of an emaciated patient. Ferguson (1961) thought that numerous large nodes were of bad prognostic import. The Aberdeen notes do not permit any definite conclusions to be drawn. It is known that some patients in whom grossly enlarged nodes were left behind in the mesentery have remained well for up to 10 years. Likewise leaving a skip area within the abdomen does not necessarily mean that the patient will have symptoms afterwards. In 12 per cent of 150 traced patients in Leeds (Atwell *et al.*, 1965) there was known to be persistent disease, yet these patients were completely asymptomatic. There is a considerable discrepancy between the doctor's rate of recurrence and the rate of invalidism as assessed by the patient (Davis, 1961). Multiple skip areas probably have the same prognostic implication as very extensive, anatomically continuous disease.

Length of Intestine Resected. This is of little value in determining prognosis. In the Aberdeen series the mean length of intestine excised in those who remained symptom-free was 59 cm. Among those who developed recurrences up to and beyond 10 years the mean length was 61 cm. These 2 groups are not strictly comparable in duration of follow-up. Furthermore, methods used by surgeons to measure the extent of their resections mostly are not stated; some values are those recorded by pathologists after fixatives have caused shrinkage of the specimen.

The Mayo Clinic workers (1954), Ferguson (1961) and Davis (1961) all have stated that the greater the extent of the disease in the intestine, the worse will be the prognosis after resection. Today patients with very extensive disease might not be submitted to resection. It has also been stated that the length of macroscopically normal intestine proximal to the lesion that is excised is unimportant. The number of accurate measurements of seemingly normal bowel included with Aberdeen specimens is small, but suggests that patients may be less likely to develop recurrence if at least 20 cm of proximal intestine is removed. Atwell *et al.* (1965) in Leeds found that when resection was "adequate" the recurrence rate was 32 per cent; when "skimped" it rose to 85 per cent. More than half their patients had been followed for over 5 years. Crohn (1955) has recommended removing at least 30 cm of intestine beyond the macroscopic upper and lower limits of the disease. Wallensten (1971) of Malmo, Sweden, also advocated radical resection.

Histology. Sixty per cent of the patients who have remained symptom-free after resection up to mid-1970 did have a granulomatous reaction, with or without giant cells, on histological examination; every patient had transmural inflammation. Among the 20 patients (out of 60 survivors) who sooner or later developed recurrent Crohn's disease, 65 per cent had a granulomatous reaction. Histological appearances are no guide to prognosis, a conclusion shared by van Patter *et al.* (1954) and Antonious *et al.* (1960). The latter authors made a detailed study of specimens from 30 patients who had been followed for at least 5 years. As well as correlating the presence of a granulomatous reaction with late results, they studied pyloric gland (Brunner-type) changes and endarteritis. Kawel and Tesluk (1955) had suggested that pyloric gland appearances heralded a gloomy clinical course, but Antonious and colleagues found no evidence to confirm this. Vascular changes had no effect on prognosis.

Late Recurrences

Four out of the 15 patients who have been followed-up for more than 10 years have developed recurrent Crohn's disease—at 12, 17, 18 and 20 years respectively after their first resection. As only a few patients have been followed for over 15 years this high incidence of late recurrence after many years of seemingly good health is disconcerting. It is recognized by all those who have carried out long-term studies (van Patter *et al.*, 1954; Crohn and Yarnis, 1958; Fielding, 1970; de Dombal *et al.*, 1971). It is probably not due to resections performed 20 years ago being insufficiently radical. The factors which originally caused the disease likely have been present all along, and by their interaction have once again caused it to appear. Hence, at the present time, it is unwise to talk of the "cure" of Crohn's disease.

Mortality in Crohn's Disease

For many years it was believed that Crohn's disease rarely killed patients suffering from it. In 1958 Crohn and Yarnis reported that the mortality for the Mount Sinai Hospital series was less than 5 per cent. Acheson (1959) obtained the tabulations of deaths in the United States, Canada, and in England and Wales for which Crohn's disease was certified as the primary cause in various years between 1950 and 1957. There were approximately 115 deaths per year from Crohn's disease in the United States. The average age-specific death rate, however, was higher in England and Wales than in the United States, being 0·11 per 100,000 and 0·08 per 100,000 respectively. There was a relative deficit among negroes and in the southern states. The death rate was higher in city dwellers compared to those living in rural areas in America, but the population of cities tends to be slightly older.

Some of the deaths in Crohn's disease are directly attributable to operations and have been discussed on page 190. The series reported by Davis (1961) consisted of 141 patients from the London area. During the review period a total of 16 died. In 13 patients (9·8 per cent) the cause of death was Crohn's disease. Davis calculated that Crohn's disease killed 1 patient out of every 750,000 people each year. During a follow-up period of from 1 to 25 years, 26 patients died (15·2 per cent) in Leeds out of a series of 172 patients (Atwell *et al.*, 1965); 15 of the deaths (8·7 per cent) were attributed to Crohn's disease. The Leeds series has now grown to 332 patients followed for over 30 years (de Dombal *et al.*, 1971); 54 patients have died (16·2 per cent), death being attributed to Crohn's disease in 41 (12·3 per cent) in the latest report. Twenty-four patients died in hospital after operation, and 30 died later. In a comparable series in Boston, also followed up for over 30 years, Banks *et al.* (1969) had an overall mortality of 14·9 per cent, while that due to Crohn's disease was 9 per cent.

Crude overall mortalities are difficult to interpret when they relate to series that have slowly accumulted over a great many years. To overcome this difficulty Prior *et al.* (1970) calculated the expectation of death by cause based on the Registrar General's statistics for the English population in 1956, the median year of the Birmingham survey. By linear interpolation they were able to derive sex and age-specific mortality rates. The experience of the 295 patients in their series was then expressed in terms of the number of individual years at risk since Crohn's disease commenced; by applying the age and sex-specific mortality rates to these results the expected number of deaths from several causes was determined. The probability of occurrence of the number of deaths actually observed, or more, was then calculated (taking the expected number as being the mean of a Poisson distribution). The actual number of deaths recorded was about twice that expected for both males and females. This was true no matter whether it was the large or the small intestine that was diseased in patients under 40 years; in older patients expected mortality rates are higher and the difference was not significant. Twenty-five out of the 53 deaths were the direct result of Crohn's disease. Among the remaining deaths there was a significant excess mortality from neoplasms of the alimentary tract, from blood diseases and from malignant hypertension compared to what would have been expected for the age and sex of the patients. Prior and her colleagues believed that the deaths from hypertension might have been contributed to by the administration of corticosteroids.

Like the Leeds and Boston series, that in Birmingham has been slowly built up for over 30 years. The Aberdeen series has only been accumulating for slightly more than 15 years. Out of 166 patients there have been 17 deaths. Only 4 out of the 60 males died compared to 13 out of 106 females (not statistically significant). The site of the disease and the use of steroids had no effect on the mortality (Table 4). The

Table 4

Effect of sex, site of disease and administration of steroids on the overall mortality of Crohn's disease

Factor	No. of patients	No. of deaths	Mortality* (per cent)
Sex: Female	106	13	12·3
Male	60	4	6·7
Site: Small Bowel	133	14	10·5
Large Bowel	33	3	9·1
Steroids: Given	64	8	12·5
Not given	102	9	8·8

* The differences between mortalities in paired factors are not statistically significant.

exact cause of death is not known for one patient. In 10 cases Crohn's disease was directly responsible, all these patients dying within 28 days of operation or perforation. In 2 other patients who developed obstruction, Crohn's disease was the probable cause. Thus there were 12 deaths attributable to Crohn's disease, giving a mortality from that condition of 7·2 per cent. One elderly female died from pneumonia and electrolyte disturbance and an elderly male from multiple lung and an unsuspected hepatic abscess; Crohn's disease may have contributed to their deaths but was not directly responsible for them. Only 2 deaths were clearly due to unrelated causes.

The crude overall mortality for the Aberdeen series is 10·2 per cent. While this percentage is about 50 per cent lower than that noted above in other series, the deaths have taken place during a much shorter follow-up period. How meaningful an overall mortality figure is remains uncertain, but the Aberdeen percentage probably indicates that the good results for resection reported on page 194 were not being achieved by adopting too strict indications for operation and debarring some ill patients from the chance of surgical relief of their symptoms. The age at onset of Crohn's disease in some of the patients may have been an important factor contributing to the mortality. Seven out of the 17 did not develop symptoms till after the age of 60 years; 3 were over 80 years old when they died. Eight deaths were the result of definitive operations, so that there was no undue reluctance to advise operation. Two patients who had had earlier laparotomies refused to have resections. The 2 deaths from perforation probably could have been avoided by timely resection.

In order to reduce the mortality, resection should be performed before the patient's condition has deteriorated too far. When it is carried out carefully, at the optimal time, and with the proper indications, primary resection for ileal disease now has a mortality of less than 2 per cent. It allows 2 out of 3 patients to enjoy 10 years or more of useful and active life, free from the restrictions, inconvenience and dangers of prolonged medical therapy.

References

Acheson, E. D. (1959), *J. Chronic Dis.*, **10**, 481.
Antonius, J. I., Gump, F. E., Lattes, R. and Lepore, M. (1960), *Gastroenterology*, **38**, 889.
Atwell, J. D., Duthie, H. L. and Goligher, J. C. (1965), *Brit. J. Surg.*, **52**, 966.
Banks, B. M., Zetzel, L. and Richter, H. S. (1969), *Amer. J. Digest. Dis.*, **14**, 369.
Best, C. N. (1959), *Brit. med. J.*, **2**, 862.
Brill, C. B., Klein, S. F. and Kark, A. E. (1969), *Ann. Surg.*, **170**, 759.
Burman, H., Williams, J. A. and Cooke, W. T. (1970), *Gut*, **11**, 1066.
Burton, I., de Dombal, F. T. and Goligher, J. C. (1969), *Brit. J. Surg.*, **56**, 692.
Cooke, W. T. (1955), *Ann. Roy. Coll. Surg. Engl.*, **17**, 137.
Chen, K. M. (1969), *Surgery*, **65**, 931.
Colcock, B. P. and Vansant, J. H. (1960), *Lahey Clin. Bull.*, **12**, 53.
Cornes, J. S. and Stecher, M. (1961), *Gut*, **2**, 189.
Crismer, R. and Dreze, C. (1962), *Rev. Med. Liege*, **17**, 709.
Crohn, B. B. (1955), *J. Mt. Sinai Hosp.*, **22**, 143.
Crohn, B. B. and Yarnis, H. (1958), *Regional Ileitis*, 2nd Edition. New York: Grune & Stratton.
Davis, J. M. (1961), *Postgrad. Med. J.*, **37**, 783.
de Dombal, F. T. (1968), *Gut*, **9**, 144.
de Dombal, F. T., Burton, I. and Goligher, J. C. (1971a), *Gut*, **12**, 519.
de Dombal, F. T., Burton, I. and Goligher, J. C. (1971b), *Brit. J. Surg.*, **58**, 805.
Doak, P. B., Montgomerie, J. Z., North, J. D. K., and Smith, F. (1968), *Brit. med. J.*, **4**, 746.
Farmer, R. G., Hawk, W. A. and Turnbull, R. B. (1968), *Amer. J. Digest. Dis.*, **13**, 501.

Ferguson, L. K. (1961), *New Engl. J. Med.*, **264**, 748.
Fielding, J. F. (1970), M.D. Thesis, National University of Ireland.
Garlock, J. H. and Crohn, B. B. (1945), *J. Amer. med. Ass.*, **127**, 205.
Goldstein, M. J., Schacter, H. and Kirsner, J. B. (1968), *Amer. J. Surg.*, **115**, 376.
Gump, F. and Lepore, M. (1960), *Gastroenterology*, **39**, 694.
Gupta, R. S., Chatterjee, A. K., Roy, R. and Ghosh, B. N. (1962), *Indian J. Surg.*, **24**, 797.
Heaton, L. D. (1964), *Ann. Surg.*, **159**, 661.
Hill, A. B. (1966), *Principles of Medical Statistics*. 8th Edition. London: Lancet.
Hughes, C. W., Baugh, J. H., Mologne, L. A. and Heaton, L. D. (1971), *Ann. Surg.*, **173**, 793.
Jones, J. H. and Lennard-Jones, J. E. (1966), *Gut*, **7**, 181.
Kawel, C. A. and Tesluk, H. (1955), *Gastroenterology*, **28**, 810.
Kent, T. H., Ammon, R. K. and Den Beston, L. (1970), *Arch. Path.*, **89**.
Kiefer, E. D. (1955), *Surg. Clin. N. Amer.*, **35**, 801.
Kipping, R. A. (1970), *Proc. Roy. Soc. Med.* **63**, 753.
Korelitz, B. I. (1967), *Gut*, **8**, 281.
Kyle, J. (1971), *Brit. J. Surg.*, **58**, 735.
Latchis, K. S., Rao, C. S. and Colcock, B. P. (1971), *Amer. J. Surg.*, **121**, 418.
Lennard-Jones, J. E. and Stalder, G. A. (1967), *Gut*, **8**, 332.
Lewin, K. and Swales, J. D. (1966), *Gastroenterology*, **50**, 211.
Marshak, R. H., Linder, A. E. and Janowitz, H. D. (1966), *Gut*, **7**, 258.
Patterson, J. F., Norton, R. A. and Schwartz, R. S. (1971), *Amer. J. Digest. Dis.*, **16**, 327.
Prior, P., Fielding, J. F., Waterhouse, J. A. and Cooke, W. T. (1970), *Lancet*, **2**, 1135.
Slaney, G. (1968), *Brit. med. J.*, **3**, 294.
Sparberg, M. and Kirsner, J. B. (1966), *Amer. J. Digest. Dis.*, **11**, 865.
Stahlgren, L. H. and Ferguson, L. K. (1961), *J. Amer. med. Ass.*, **175**, 986.
Truelove, S. C. (1971), in *Regional Enteritis (Crohn's Disease)*. Edit. A. Engel and T. Larsson. Stockholm: Skandia International Symposia.
van Patter, W. N., Bargen, J. A., Dockerty, M. B., Feldman, W. H., Mayo, C. W. and Waugh, J. M. (1954), *Gastroenterology*, **26**, 347.
Wallensten, S. (1971), in *Regional Enteritis (Crohn's Disease)*. Edit. A. Engel and T. Larsson. Stockholm: Skandia International Symposia.
Windsor, C. W. O., Fejfar, J. and Woodward, D. A. K. (1969), *Gut*, **10**, 779.
Yarnis, H. and Crohn, B. B. (1960), *Gastroenterology*, **38**, 721.

Index